Instructor's Manual for

Black and Matassarin-Jacobs

Medical-Surgical Nursing

Clinical Management for Continuity of Care

Fifth Edition

Elizabeth Ann Coleman, PhD, RNP, AOCN
Professor
College of Nursing
University of Arkansas for Medical Sciences
Little Rock, Arkansas

Janet E. Lord, PhD, RN
Associate Professor
Chair, Adult Health Department
College of Nursing
University of Arkansas for Medical Sciences
Little Rock, Arkansas

Sue Wyatt Huskey, MSN, RN, CCRN
Clinical Assistant Professor
College of Nursing
University of Arkansas for Medical Sciences
Little Rock, Arkansas

W.B. SAUNDERS COMPANY
A Division of Harcourt Brace & Company
Philadelphia London Toronto Montreal Sydney Tokyo

W.B. SAUNDERS COMPANY
A Division of Harcourt Brace & Company
The Curtis Center
Independence Square West
Philadelphia, Pennsylvania 19106-3399

Instructor's Manual for Black and Matassarin-Jacobs
MEDICAL-SURGICAL NURSING
Clinical Management for Continuity of Care, 5th Edition

ISBN 0–7216–6400–8

Printed in the United States of America.

Last digit is the print number: 9 8 7 6 5 4 3 2 1

Dedications

To the nurses in my family: my daughter, Janine Roxanne Jones, my mother, Ouida Lee Griffith Brett, and my sister, Glenda Joyce Rainer, and to my husband, Lawrence, for his constant love, support, and encouragement.

Ann Coleman

To my father, Vayne Lord, and my special brother, Michael Wayne Lord, for their love and support.

Janet Lord

To my husband, Harold, and my children Brian and Melissa for helping me keep the important things in perspective, my parents Wayne and Olivia Wyatt for their encouragement and support, and my sister Carol Wyatt Dean, the other nurse in the family.

Sue Huskey

Preface

This *Instructor's Manual* was developed to accompany **Medical-Surgical Nursing: Clinical Management for Continuity of Care,** 5th Edition, edited by Joyce Black and Esther Matassarin-Jacobs. It is intended to assist nursing instructors with ideas for teaching in the classroom and clinical areas. Because teaching styles vary, it is not expected that all the activities suggested will be appropriate for any one teacher. The experienced teacher may use the suggestions to expand his or her repertoire of teaching techniques. For the beginning teacher, the suggestions may provide a framework for presenting content as well as some useful aids, like the transparencies. It also provides suggestions for clinical activities and postconferences that will clarify classroom material for students.

The chapters are organized with student learning objectives, review activities, specific ideas for lecture/discussions, suggestions for group activities, and guest lecturers in the classroom. Clinical learning experience suggestions are coordinated with classroom topics to assist student transfer of knowledge to the clinical area. The clinical suggestions include skills laboratory, clinical site, and clinical conference activities. Some of the chapters contain a "Critical Points to Emphasize" section.

Case studies are included in some chapters of the *Study Guide.* These can be used in classroom teaching or postconference to teach care of clients with specific disorders. Additional case studies are presented in the textbook. The clinical commentaries (Appendix A in the *Study Guide*) on these cases will help students transfer knowledge from the clinical setting in school to the clinical setting in practice. Questions from the *Study Guide* can also be used to facilitate class or clinical conference discussions and help students prepare for examinations.

Appendixes B, C, and D in the *Study Guide* contain forms for worksheets for organizing information on the classical/textbook picture of any disorder, note-taking outlines/worksheets for arrhythmias, and blank grids for gathering data. These worksheets will help students focus their learning in the clinical setting.

Over 150 four-color transparencies were developed to go along with textbook materials. The *Instructor's Manual* refers to specific transparencies for each chapter of the text from the color transparencies kit *Transparencies to Accompany Luckmann's Core Principles and Practice of Medical-Surgical Nursing* ***and*** *Luckmann's Medical-Surgical Nursing,* fifth edition. These word and diagram transparencies will be useful in small or large classrooms to enhance both teaching and learning.

The disk accompanying the *Study Guide* contains questions in the NCLEX format with answers and rationales. There are test-taking tips specific to some questions. The questions are referred to by unit, chapter, and topic in the text. We hope our ideas and suggestions for ways to facilitate teaching will be helpful.

Acknowledgments

We offer thanks to the individuals who helped us with this *Instructor's Manual.*

To Norma L. Pinnell, MSN, RN, faculty member with the Colleges of Nursing at Southern Illinois University at Edwardsville in Edwardsville, IL and Deaconess Health System in St. Louis, MO, who was one of the authors (along with Ann and Janet) of the third and fourth editions of the *Instructor's Manual for Luckmann and Sorensen's Medical-Surgical Nursing: A Psychophysiologic Approach.* Her valuable contributions are a part of the current work.

To Sharon K. Coon, MNSc, RN, AOCN, a fellow faculty member with us in the College of Nursing at the University of Arkansas for Medical Sciences in Little Rock, AR, who helped Ann prepare the *Study Disk* accompanying the *Study Guide.* The disk contains questions in the NCLEX format with answers and rationales.

To each of the clinical experts who wrote clinical commentaries for the case studies presented in the textbook **Medical-Surgical Nursing: Clinical Management for Continuity of Care,** 5th Edition by Black and Matassarin-Jacobs. The clinical commentaries are presented in the Appendix of the *Study Guide.*

To Lisa King, Editorial & Production Services, who helped design and prepare the final manuscript for production.

To Elizabeth Byrd, Associate Developmental Editor, who provided support and encouragement and helped keep us on schedule during manuscript preparation and editing.

To Thomas Eoyang, Vice-President & Editor-in-Chief, Nursing Books, who supervised the acquisition and overall production of the ancillary package.

To Melanie Nordlinger, former Editorial Assistant, who served as interim "developmental editor" and kept the chapters from the textbook coming and supported us during manuscript preparation.

Contents

Unit IV Immunologic Disorders

Unit V Neurologic Disorders

Unit VI Eye and Ear Disorders

Unit VII Respiratory Disorders

Unit VIII Cardiac Disorders

Unit IX Peripheral Vascular Disorders

Unit X Hematologic Disorders

Unit XI Urinary Disorders

Unit XII Gastrointestinal Disorders

Unit XIII Liver, Biliary Tract, and Exocrine Pancreatic Disorders

Unit XIV Metabolic Disorders

CHAPTER

1

The Context of Medical-Surgical Nursing

Objectives

1.1 Discuss the major groups and institutions involved in the United States healthcare system.

1.2 Describe the various mechanisms available for funding healthcare.

1.3 Discuss the major focuses of the Period of Expansion, the Period of Regulation and Cost Containment, and the Period of Reform.

1.4 List settings in which the nurse practices today.

1.5 Describe four of the special client populations that nurses serve.

1.6 Discuss the American Nurses' Association's (ANA's) role in healthcare reform.

Facilitating Student Learning

CLASSROOM

Class Assignments

- Assign chapter in study guide.
- Have students identify one health-related legislation currently being considered in their state.
- Ask students to interview an individual on a governing board of a local hospital to determine their role in the healthcare system.
- Ask students to interview four healthcare consumers to determine their concerns with the present healthcare system. Share these findings in a classroom discussion.

Lecture/Discussion

- Discuss the stakeholders in the U.S. healthcare system.
- Discuss the evolution of funding programs in the United States. Describe the events that occurred during the Period of Expansion and the Period of Regulation and Cost Containment.
- Discuss the Period of Healthcare Reform.
- Review Box 1–1, Funding Programs, with students.
- Share highlights from *Nursing's Agenda for Health Care Reform* with students.
- Discuss the *Healthy People 2000: An Overview of the National Health Promotion and Disease Prevention Objectives* report.
- Discuss the ANA's role in healthcare reform.

Guest Speakers

- Ask a nurse lobbyist to describe the legislative role of nurses.
- Have a panel of nurses from various care settings describe their roles.

Group Activities

- Divide the class into small groups. Ask each group to identify and discuss factors that affect the healthcare delivery system.
- Divide the class into small groups. Ask each group to discuss the implications of the changing healthcare delivery system on nursing.

CLINICAL

Clinical Site Activities

- Assign students to survey the records of clients on a division to determine the sources of healthcare funding being used.
- Assign students to examine the typical length of stay in hospitals compared to 10 years ago.

Clinical Conference Activities

- Ask the person in charge of Utilization Review to speak to the students.
- Ask a nurse who has been in practice at least 15 years to discuss changes in nursing practice.

CHAPTER

2

Theories of Health and Illness

Objectives

2.1 Discuss the major theories of disease/illness and the scientists associated with each.

2.2 Discuss the relationship between mediators of stress and illness.

2.3 Explain multifactorial aspects of chronic diseases.

2.4 Describe the concepts of health and illness.

Facilitating Student Learning

CLASSROOM

Class Assignments

- Ask students to compare the homeostatic, psychosocial, and bio-behavioral theoretical bases for disease.
- Ask students to evaluate their chance of developing an illness based on Holmes' and Rahne's Social Readjustment Rating Scale.
- Ask students to describe how they handle stress in their own lives.
- Ask students to discuss how the mind-body relationship affects health and nursing practice.
- Ask students to write down what they believe causes illness.
- Assign students to ask friends and family what they believe causes illness and to be prepared to discuss the implications these beliefs have on nursing care.

Lecture/Discussion

- Focus the lecture/discussion on one example of each of the main types of theories discussed in this chapter: homeostatic, psychosocial, and bio-behavioral.
- Use Figure 2–2 to assist in the explanation of the general adaptation syndrome.
- Emphasize the physiologic and psychologic responses associated with each theory discussed.

Transparency

- 3–2(T)—The General Adaptation Syndrome (Figure 2–2)

Group Activities

- Divide class into small groups. Assign students to describe their responses to stress. Ask them to discuss the physiologic bases for their stress responses.
- Divide class into small groups. Ask students to compare how disease and illness are viewed according to the theories of Bernard and Cannon, Selye, Mason, Wolff, Lazarus, Wolf, Schwartz, and Friedman and Rosenman.

CLINICAL

Clinical Site Activities

- Assign students to collect health history and physical assessment on an individual.
- Assign students to analyze their findings according to Selye's, Schwartz's, or Lazarus' theory.

Clinical Conference Activities

- Ask students to discuss their assessment findings and the results of their analyses.
- Assign students to rate their assigned client according to the Social Readjustment Rating Scale. Ask the conference group to discuss the significance of these findings. Assign them to discuss the uses and limitations of such rating scales.

CHAPTER

3

Ethics

Objectives

3.1 Define terms associated with ethics and moral philosophy.

3.2 Identify basic principles that serve as the foundation for ethical decision-making.

3.3 Discuss the basic principles presented in the *American Nurses' Association's Code for Nurses with Interpretive Statements.*

3.4 Describe four parameters or guidelines for nursing practice.

3.5 Differentiate between the theories of deontology and teleology to guide ethical decision-making.

3.6 Compare the steps in the nursing process to those in Murphy and Murphy's ethical decision-making model.

3.7 Discuss the concepts of research and ethics.

3.8 Discuss three ethical concerns for nurses.

3.9 Discuss three ethical concerns for clients.

Facilitating Student Learning

CLASSROOM

Class Assignments

- Ask students to complete the section in Study Guide before class session.
- Assign students to write their own personal definitions for the terms *ethics* and *morals*.
- Ask students to bring to class one ethical concern related to their own experiences in nursing.

Lecture/Discussion

- Content in this chapter lends itself to discussion format and not lecture format. Students will have a better understanding of the material if they are active in the learning process.
- Discuss the definitions of key terms from the chapter. Ask students to apply knowledge from other courses that discussed ethics, e.g., philosophy courses, medical ethics course.
- Provide students with personal copies of the *American Nurses' Association's Code for Nurses with Interpretive Statements*. These are available through the ANA.
- Select several statements listed in the code and discuss them in class. Place statements on transparencies to facilitate class participation.
- Discuss the guidelines for practice presented in this chapter. Ask students to discuss how these guidelines affect their nursing practice.

Guest Speakers

- Arrange for someone from the philosophy department to discuss with the class the topic of ethical issues in nursing.
- Arrange for an attorney to talk with the class about the state's living will and durable power of attorney for healthcare laws.

Group Activity

- Divide the class into small groups; provide each group with a case study. Assign the groups to determine the ethical issue presented in their case study. Ask them to use one of the ethical decision-making models discussed in the chapter to analyze the issue. Have the groups share their analyses with the class during a discussion period.

CLINICAL

Clinical Site Activities

- Assign students to identify one ethical issue apparent in the clinical setting.
- Ask students to find the standards of care for clients on their assigned division.
- Ask students to determine what information is provided clients about the *Patients' Bill of Rights*.

Clinical Conference Activities

- Arrange for someone from the agency's ethics committee to speak to students.
- Have students consider this issue: Is healthcare a right or privilege?
- Have students discuss an ethical issue related to a client on their division.

CHAPTER

4

Psychosocial Dimensions of Medical-Surgical Nursing

Objectives

4.1 Discuss various definitions of *family*.
4.2 Identify common family structures found in the United States.
4.3 Discuss the functions of a family.
4.4 Discuss the five levels of family functioning according to Tapia and their implications for nursing care.
4.5 Complete a family assessment including a genogram.
4.6 Discuss potential nursing interventions for the client and family during the illness experience.
4.7 Differentiate between culture and cultural diversity.
4.8 Discuss terminology related to cross-cultural nursing.
4.9 Discuss the two main theories of health and illness.
4.10 Examine personal beliefs in relation to the concept of cultural sensitivity.
4.11 Perform a cultural assessment.
4.12 Discuss the concept of international nursing.
4.13 Differentiate between spirituality and religion.
4.14 Discuss the implications of client spirituality for your nursing care.
4.15 Discuss the psychosocial and sociocultural elements of sexuality.
4.16 Describe the nurse's roles in promoting sexual health.
4.17 Perform a sexual assessment.
4.18 Discuss applications for the PLISSIT Model for Sexual Health Interventions.
4.19 Discuss the impact of illness on sexuality.

Facilitating Student Learning

CLASSROOM

Class Assignments

- Assign students to develop their personal definitions of family and compare their personal definitions to the inclusive definition in their text.
- Assign students to complete a cultural assessment on a classmate and identify appropriate nursing diagnoses and interventions.
- Ask students to identify ethnic groups and subcultures within their communities.
- Assign students to write a one-page paper expanding on the similarities and differences of spirituality and religion.
- Assign students to examine their beliefs and concerns about aspects of human sexuality.

Lecture/Discussion

- Content in this chapter lends itself to discussion rather than lecture format. Students will gain a better understanding of their own beliefs relevant to the psychosocial dimensions of nursing if they are active in the learning process.
- Using a family assessment, construct a genogram with the students.
- From the students' comparisons of definitions of family, lead a class discussion on how to provide care to clients whose families are different from the students'.
- Have students identify and discuss how non-Western health practices could be included in their plan of care.
- Guide a student discussion on when to complete a spiritual assessment, components of a spiritual assessment, and nursing interventions for a nursing diagnosis of spiritual distress.
- Discuss areas of student concerns in working with issues related to human sexuality.
- Invite a guest speaker experienced in values clarification to work with students on recognizing their personal values, how they may be in conflict with their clients' values, and identifying ways of managing these differences.
- Apply the PLISSIT Model for Sexual Health Interventions to the situation of a 34-year-old man postop abdominal-perineal resection for colon cancer.

Group Activity

- Have students role play obtaining a family history.

CLINICAL

Clinical Site Activities

- Assign students to conduct a family assessment on their assigned client, analyze the family structure and level of functioning, develop nursing diagnoses, and identify appropriate interventions.
- Assign students to complete cultural assessments on their clients and develop nursing diagnoses and interventions.
- Assign students to assess clients for spiritual distress and identify appropriate nursing diagnoses and interventions.
- Assign students to obtain sexual histories on their clients.

Clinical Conference Activities

- Assign students to seek information on support services, visiting hours, and nursing service philosophy statements in relation to families in the hospital where they are completing their clinical rotations. Discuss the students' findings in postconference.
- Assign a student with a client whose actual nursing diagnosis is Altered family coping or ineffective family coping to lead a postconference on the care of the client and family.

- Assign students to bring a current journal article to conference that contains research on or discussion of cross-cultural nursing.
- Have students examine nutrition practices of various religions. Discuss with students their findings and how these practices may differ from usual hospital routine and treatment regimens. Problem-solve with students on ways to meet the client's needs and medical treatments.

CHAPTER

5

Aging

OBJECTIVES

5.1 Define terminology related to aging.

5.2 Discuss demographics related to persons over 65.

5.3 Discuss health promotion activities for persons over 65.

5.4 Describe physiologic and psychosocial factors influencing functional status of elderly persons.

5.5 Compare and contrast dementia, delirium, and depression.

5.6 Discuss medication use and abuse among persons over 65.

5.7 Describe government support, healthcare resources, services, and housing options for persons over 65.

5.8 Discuss ethical and legal issues affecting persons over 65.

Facilitating Student Learning

CLASSROOM

Class Assignments

- Have students interview a person over 65 to identify physical, psychosocial, and health issues which are of concern.
- Assign students to obtain a copy of one of the instruments used for measuring functional status.
- Assign students to explore housing options for persons over 65 available in their community.
- Assign students to visit a community agency serving persons over 65 to determine what services are provided and how nurses can direct clients to these services.

Lecture/Discussion

- This chapter content lends itself to discussion rather than lecture format.
- Lead a class discussion on the impact that the number of persons over 65 will have on nursing and the healthcare industry by 2020 and 2030.
- Discuss with students the issue of rationing of healthcare.
- Lead a discussion of stereotypes applied to persons over 65. Discuss measures nurses can use in their care of clients to overcome these negative stereotypes.
- Discuss community agencies and government programs that provide services for persons over 65.
- Discuss major health issues for persons over 65.
- Have students report on their findings regarding housing options available in their community. Lead a discussion of the students' findings on the adequacy of the housing options and make recommendations for changes.
- Have students report on their findings about community agencies providing services for persons over 65.

Guest Speaker

- Invite a person from the American Association of Retired Persons (AARP) to discuss legislation of potential benefit to persons over 65 which is or is not being supported.

CLINICAL

Clinical Site Activities

- Assign students to clients over 65. Have students complete one of the functional assessment instruments. From these data and data from a completed health assessment, have students focus on actual or potential alterations in activities of daily living (ADLs) or instrumental activities of daily living (IADLs) and interventions.
- Have students use data from their assessment to analyze their clients' medication patterns (prescriptions and OTC). Have students discuss drug interactions, client understanding of medication purpose, and ability to comply with medical regimen. Work with students to identify actual or potential nursing diagnoses and interventions.
- Again using data from the students' assessments, have students analyze their clients' nutrition and develop actual or potential nursing diagnoses and interventions.
- As part of their nursing care plans have students develop and implement a teaching plan for their clients that includes applicable teaching principles for persons over 65.

Clinical Conference Activity

- Use postconference as a forum for students to discuss and analyze their clients' actual or potential nursing diagnoses and interventions related to ADLs, IADLs, medications, and nutrition. Invite a faculty member whose specialty is gerontology to consult with students.

CHAPTER

6

Chronic Conditions

Objectives

6.1 Discuss general concepts related to chronic conditions.

6.2 Discuss the processes of adaptation as they relate to chronic conditions.

6.3 Describe various healthcare facilities that provide care for persons with chronic conditions.

6.4 Describe nursing management for clients with chronic conditions.

Facilitating Student Learning

CLASSROOM

Class Assignments

- Assign students to answer the questions in the Study Guide.
- Assign students to visit a facility that focuses on care of persons with chronic illnesses. Have students identify the unit's philosophy regarding care of persons with chronic illnesses and how these beliefs are implemented.

Lecture/Discussion

- Discuss the importance of the nurse's role in preventing complications for the hospitalized client with a chronic condition.
- To help students appreciate the impact of a chronic condition, ask students to share personal experiences with chronic conditions.
- Discuss with students differences they may see between the sick role behaviors of clients with chronic conditions and those with acute conditions.
- Lead students in a discussion of physiologic, psychologic, and sociologic adaptive changes and challenges that persons with chronic conditions may face.
- Discuss with students the effect of a chronic condition on the family.
- Have students share their observations and assessments of facilities that focus on care of persons with chronic illnesses.
- Discuss with students nursing care for clients in the various stages of, and with various types of, chronic conditions.

CLINICAL

Clinical Site Activities

- Assign students to a client with a chronic condition. Assist them in selecting one or more of the assessment tools identified in the textbook and using it to assess their client's status.
- Assign students to identify nursing diagnoses and interventions based on the assessments.
- Have students identify specific education needs for their clients and families based on their assessments.

Clinical Conference Activities

- In postconference, select one student to present the database on his or her client with a chronic condition. Guide group discussion around topics of stage of client's adaptation to illness, client and family coping behaviors, role changes in the family necessitated by the condition, rehabilitation potential, and community services that might be needed by the client and/or family.
- Invite a person with a chronic condition to come to postconference to discuss the effect of the condition on his or her life, coping strategies, community resources, role changes, rehabilitation, and family.
- Invite a representative from a community agency to come to postconference and describe the services that are available through that agency for persons with chronic conditions.

CHAPTER

7

Acute Care

Objectives

7.1 Discuss the historical changes that have occurred in relation to hospital nursing.

7.2 Describe hospital facilities available for clients who require acute care and subacute care.

7.3 Describe roles and responsibilities of nurses in hospitals.

7.4 Compare and contrast nursing care delivery systems.

7.5 Discuss the role of the licensed nurse in managing unlicensed assistive personnel.

7.6 Discuss various measures whose purposes are to ensure quality healthcare delivery.

Facilitating Student Learning

CLASSROOM

Class Assignments

- Assign students to interview a hospital staff nurse who has been in the acute care setting for at least 10 years to elicit a personal account of changes that have occurred and continue to occur in the setting.
- Assign students to investigate one of the measures identified in the textbook for assuring quality of healthcare delivery.

Lecture/Discussion

- Content in this chapter lends itself to discussion format.
- Discuss with students the various roles of the nurse in an acute care setting.
- Summarize for students the changes occurring in healthcare and their impact on hospital nursing as background for discussion of the results of students' interviews with staff nurses.
- Have students complete a 3–5 minute presentation on the measure they investigated for assuring quality of healthcare delivery.
- Divide students into teams to debate the pros and cons of the various nursing care delivery systems.
- Share with students the Nurse Practice Act rules and regulations for delegating tasks to unlicensed assistive personnel.

Guest Speakers

- Invite a nursing service administrator to discuss the changes occurring in hospitals and nursing service.
- Invite a risk manager to discuss his/her role.
- Invite a nurse who manages the hospital accreditation reviews to discuss their purposes, processes, outcomes, and costs.

CLINICAL

Clinical Site Activities

- Assign students to identify the nursing care delivery system used on the unit to which they are assigned.
- Have students work with a staff nurse to complete the nursing intensity classification.
- Have each student investigate the roles and responsibilities of one of the support service departments in the hospital.

Clinical Conference Activities

- Have students report the results of their investigation of one of the support service departments.
- Review with students the nursing intensity classification results. Did the system outcomes match the student's perception of the level of care required for the client? Did the system identify a staffing level which matched the student's perception of the unit's needs?

CHAPTER

8

Ambulatory Care

Objectives

8.1 Define the terms related to ambulatory care.

8.2 Discuss the major changes in healthcare that have resulted in an increase in ambulatory care services.

8.3 Discuss the general discharge criteria for ambulatory care.

8.4 Discuss the role of the nurse in ambulatory care.

Facilitating Student Learning

CLASSROOM

Class Assignment

- Ask students to complete the section in the Study Guide before class session.

Lecture/Discussion

- Content in this chapter lends itself to discussion format rather than lecture format.
- Begin the discussion with a brief overview of the shift from hospital-based nursing to ambulatory care nursing.
- Discuss ambulatory care settings in your area. Ask the students to list some of the advantages of using the ambulatory settings.

Group Activities

- Divide the students into small groups and have them describe the differences in hospital nursing, home health nursing, and ambulatory care nursing.
- Provide case studies of different types of surgeries and procedures, and ask the students to choose the ones that could be performed in an ambulatory care setting. Use the two common features of ambulatory care settings on page 137 as a guide.

CLINICAL

Clinical Site Activity

- Assign students to an ambulatory care setting. Have them assess the organization of the nursing care, the use of the nursing process, and discharge criteria for the setting.

Clinical Conference Activities

- Ask students to share their experiences in the clinical setting.
- Ask students to compare and contrast ambulatory care nursing with hospital-based nursing.
- Ask the students to describe discharge criteria for their clients.
- Invite a nurse from ambulatory care to discuss the cost of services in ambulatory care settings versus hospital settings.

CHAPTER

9

Home Healthcare

Objectives

9.1 Discuss one major trend that affects home healthcare.

9.2 Discuss the eligibility, requirements, and coverage for Medicare and Medicaid.

9.3 Discuss the basic principle of community-based nursing care.

9.4 Discuss the purpose of the Omaha System of providing nursing care.

Facilitating Student Learning

CLASSROOM

Class Assignments

- Read Chapter 9.
- Ask students to complete the section in the Study Guide.

Lecture/Discussion

- Begin class by asking the question "What does 'healthcare is shifting from acute care to community-based settings' mean to you?" Summarize the students' responses.
- Give an overview of the major trends that affect the shift toward community-based settings.
- Compare and contrast nursing care in hospital-based settings and community-based settings.

Guest Speakers

- Invite a panel of representatives from various community settings to give a brief overview of their settings.

CLINICAL

Clinical Site Activities

- Assign students to a home health setting.
- Ask the students how the nursing process is used in the home health setting.
- Determine eligibility, requirements, and coverage for the client who needs home healthcare.
- Ask the student to assess the nursing roles in home healthcare.

Clinical Conference Activities

- Ask students to share their experiences in home healthcare.
- Ask students to compare and contrast nursing roles in home healthcare with nursing roles in hospital/acute care settings.

CHAPTER

10

Health Promotion

Objectives

10.1 Define terms associated with health promotion.

10.2 Describe the concept of wellness as viewed by Dunn and Travis.

10.3 Summarize the evolution of the concept of health promotion.

10.4 Explain Pender's model of health promotion.

10.5 Discuss the three levels of prevention and the behaviors associated with each level.

10.6 Identify the six categories of risk factors.

10.7 Identify three social problems that affect health and well-being.

10.8 Describe the impact of environment on health and wellness.

10.9 Discuss the relationship among nutrition, exercise, and health promotion.

10.10 Describe three methods of managing stress.

10.11 Discuss health promotion and the older adult.

Facilitating Student Learning

CLASSROOM

Review Activity

- Suggest that students review the section in Chapter 3 on stress theory.

Class Assignments

- Assign students to find three primary, secondary, and tertiary prevention measures being implemented in their community.
- Ask the students to make a list of their own healthy and unhealthy lifestyle patterns.
- Assign selected students to gather information regarding meditation, hypnosis, and self-hypnosis programs available in their community.
- Assign students to complete the food diary form in the textbook (Figure 10–7). Have them analyze the data according to the seven guidelines for a healthful diet.
- Assign students a journal article summary on some aspect of *Healthy People 2000.*

Lecture/Discussion

- Chapter 10 is short and easy to read. Discussion and clarification of content should be used instead of lecture. Allow students the opportunity to share their ideas.
- Discuss the role of the nurse in Dunn's model, Travis's model, and Pender's model.
- Provide the class with several brief scenarios about clients. Ask the students to determine where each client belongs on Travis's wellness model.
- Discuss what health promotion measures should be taught in the acute care setting; e.g., testicular examinations, self breast examination (SBE), smoking cessation.
- Although not specifically discussed in this chapter, it would be appropriate to introduce the students to the health belief model and health promotion model.

Transparencies

- Wellness Model (Figure 10–2)
- Health Promotion Model (Figure 10–3)

Group Activities

- Divide the class into small groups. Ask each group to discuss the following questions:
  - —What is holistic nursing?
  - —What are the advantages and drawbacks of a holistic approach to the nursing process?
  - —Is a policy of holistic nursing reasonable for a healthcare facility?
- Divide the class into small groups. Ask each group to discuss the question: Do persons have an obligation to avoid activities known to cause illness that, in turn, may burden society?
- Assign students to divide into pairs. Ask one student to practice a relaxation exercise while the other student monitors his/her pulse and respiratory rate.

Guest Speaker

- Ask a community health nurse to discuss health promotion and levels of prevention from the perspective of community health nursing.

CLINICAL

Clinical Site Activities

- Assign students to observe a care setting for evidence of holistic care.
- Assign students to determine their client's health promotion practices.
- Ask students to place their client on Travis's wellness model.
- Ask students to identify stressors that their client is or has been experiencing.
- Assign students to assess their client according to the food diary form in the textbook (Figure 10–7). Have them analyze the data according to the seven guidelines for a healthful diet.

Clinical Conference Activities

- Ask students to discuss observations of holistic care.
- Ask students to share assessment findings regarding stressors. Ask the conference group to discuss how these stressors might affect the client.

Critical Points to Emphasize

- *Health* is defined by the World Health Organization (WHO) as "a state of complete physical, mental, and social well-being and not merely the absence of disease or infirmity."
- *Wellness* incorporates positive mental, physical, and spiritual well-being.
- *Health promotion* is the process of fostering awareness, influencing attitudes, and identifying alternatives so individuals can make informed choices.
- *Self responsibility* is developing the awareness and ability to take action to achieve or maintain individual freedom, health, and well-being.
- *Risk factors* are genetic, environmental, or lifestyle factors that increase the probability of developing an illness or disease.
- *Community* is defined by the WHO as "a social group determined by geographic boundaries and/or common values and interests."
- Americans are more aware of health promotion and are moving toward a greater independence in the self-care role.
- Dunn was the first person to define and describe *wellness*, an idea that was a precursor to the health promotion movement.
- Dunn's high-level wellness is "an integrated method of functioning which is oriented toward maximizing the potential of which the individual is capable within the environment he is functioning."
- Dunn's work may have been stimulated by the work of Sigerist, a medical historian and the first person to describe health promotion as one of the four functions of medicine: health promotion, prevention of illness, restoration of health, and rehabilitation.
- The objective of Travis's wellness model is to demonstrate how people can move from the point of illness or neutrality into the realm of high-level wellness, and reduce the occurrence or recurrence of illness and disease.
- *Healthy People 2000* has promoted agencies to focus on prevention and promotion through strategies of institutional change, legislation, and public policy, and not merely the realm of personal behavior change.
- Nurses need to understand the underlying concepts of health promotion and illness prevention.
- Health promotion and illness prevention should be addressed in every aspect of care and in every setting.
- Level of prevention:
  - —*Primary prevention* is concerned with health promotion activities that prevent the actual occurrence of a specific illness or disease.
  - —*Secondary prevention* refers to health behaviors that promote the early detection (screening) and treatment of disease and limitation of disability.

(Continued)

Critical Points to Emphasize

(Concluded)

— *Tertiary prevention* is directed toward rehabilitation after a disease or condition has already developed.

- Risk factors are the key to health promotion. It is possible to uncover one or more risk factors during assessment.
- Nurses need to develop a method of obtaining information that achieves two goals. One goal is to obtain the most information about the presenting problem or reason the person is seeking healthcare. The second goal is to obtain information on health promotion and illness prevention. (Please refer to chapter two of Jarvis' *Physical Examination and Health Assessment* by W.B. Saunders for more information.)

CHAPTER

11

Health Assessment

Objectives

11.1 Describe the concept of health assessment.

11.2 Discuss the main components of the health history interview.

11.3 Discuss the importance of psychosocial assessment for clients with medical-surgical problems.

11.4 Discuss the eight psychosocial risk factors.

11.5 Explain the purpose of the review of symptoms and symptoms analysis portion of the physical health interview.

11.6 Record health assessment findings using an organized format.

11.7 Apply the nursing process to health assessment.

Facilitating Student Learning

CLASSROOM

Class Assignments

- Ask students to make a list of their own healthy and unhealthy lifestyle patterns.
- Assign selected students to gather information regarding screening and preventive measures available to clients in their community.
- Assign students to conduct a health history interview on a family member. Request that they include the sociologic and physical health history components.

Lecture/Discussion

- Chapter 11 provides information that students can use as reference or resource material. Testing should be on broad concepts within the chapter. Application of knowledge will occur in the clinical setting.
- Discuss the concepts of stereotyping and health assessment. Ask the students to discuss how stereotyping can be avoided.
- Discuss how the healthcare provider can assist the client assume self-care behavior in the areas of screening and prevention of disease.
- Discuss what health promotion measures are associated with each of the risk factor categories.
- Discuss health risk appraisal across the lifespan. Ask the students to give examples of risk factors associated with each age group.
- Discuss the psychosocial, sociologic, and physical health history. Provide students with examples of completed health histories.
- Role play a complete health history interview with another faculty member.

Group Activities

- Divide the class into pairs. Provide each pair with the health history form used in your program and allow them time to conduct a health history interview.

CLINICAL

Clinical Site Activity

- Assign students to conduct a health history interview on their assigned client. Remember that the complete health history may be lengthy. You may want to allow the students more than one session with the client for their initial interview. Remind students to review the example of the health history assessment in Table 11-5.

Clinical Conference Activites

- Ask students to discuss what should be done with confidential information.
- Ask students to share health history assessment findings. Have the conference group discuss how this information affects nursing care.
- The nursing process hinges on thorough assessment of the client, which provides baseline data.

Critical Points to Emphasize

- Assessment requires both skill and judgment.
- The nurse must be familiar with parameters of human behavior and physiology before being able to recognize abnormal situations.
- Health assessment requires extensive practice.
- Health assessment focuses on the individual client. The health assessment includes the health history and physical examination. The health history contains subjective information, whereas the physical examination contains objective information.
- The depth of the health history depends on the reason the person is seeking healthcare. An in-depth health history allows for a thorough assessment. An episodic health history is used to collect data about a specific problem.
- Guidelines for the health history interview include preparation of the environment, client, and interviewer.
- Components of the health history are: biographic and demographic information, physical health history: chief complaint, symptom analysis, past medical history, family history, psychosocial history, and review of systems.
- The health promotion and health risk appraisal examine risk factors that affect the client's potential for developing a particular health problem.
- Risk factors are genetic or biologic, behavioral, or environmental.
- Nurses should be aware of risk factors for individuals and groups of individuals. Developing a risk profile on every client is a good way to incorporate health promotion and illness prevention activities.
- Screen tests and procedures are used to assess if a client has a health problem or is at risk for future health problems.
- The health history is organized to obtain the maximum amount of information in the shortest time and with the fewest questions.
- There are several ways to organize the health history. Two common frameworks are the medical model and Gordon's functional health patterns.
- The medical model consists of the same areas that physicians use to gather data: biographical and demographic information, chief complaint, past medical history, family medical history, psychosocial history, and review of systems. However, nurses may include more questions about health promotion, psychosocial assessment, nutrition, spiritual assessment, and functional status to determine the client's response to health problems.
- Gordon's functional health patterns include information on the client's lifestyle, and behaviors to promote, maintain, and restore health and well-being, and review systems-type questions for each pattern.
- An advantage of the modified medical model is that it is organized in the same way physicians and other healthcare providers gather information. Thus, it may facilitate communication with other healthcare providers. An advantage of the functional health patterns is the organization of data in clusters that facilitate identifying problems and planning care.
- Nurses need to be efficient in recording the health history on agency forms and writing a narrative health history.
- The nurse uses the subjective data from the health history and objective data from the physical examination and laboratory and diagnostic tests to make judgments about the client's health status.

CHAPTER

12

Physical Examination

Objectives

12.1 Discuss the purpose of a physical examination.

12.2 Describe the types of physical examinations.

12.3 Describe the four primary techniques used in a physical examination.

12.4 Define anatomic terms used to describe locations of physical findings.

12.5 Calculate ideal body weight.

12.6 Identify equipment commonly used in a physical examination.

12.7 Discuss the preparation for a physical examination.

12.8 Demonstrate a basic adult screening physical examination.

12.9 Demonstrate ability to process and record data.

Facilitating Student Learning

CLASSROOM

CLASS ASSIGNMENTS

- Ask students to complete the section in the Study Guide before class session.
- Assign readings from the textbook, Jarvis, C. (1996). *Physical Examination and Health Assessment*, Philadelphia: W. B. Saunders, to supplement material in the chapter.

LECTURE/DISCUSSION

- Chapter 12 provides information that students can use as reference or resource material. Testing should be on broad concepts within the chapter, e.g., positions, equipment, definition of terms. Application of knowledge will occur in the clinical setting.
- Discuss the overall sequence of the physical examination. Focus on familiarizing the students with terms.

CLINICAL

SKILLS LABORATORY

- Have students examine and manipulate physical examination equipment.
- Demonstrate the general adult screening physical examination on another faculty member.
- Have students practice using selected items of equipment under the supervision of an instructor.
- Ask students to identify the following: otoscope, ophthalmoscope, oto-ophthalmoscope, nasal speculum, vaginal speculum, Snellen chart, sphygmomanometer, stethoscope, reflex hammer, and tuning fork.
- Have students practice performing a physical examination following the procedure outlined in Chapter 12. Validate their findings.
- Ask students to record assessment findings. Critique these findings and discuss with students the significance of the data.

CLINICAL SITE ACTIVITIES

- Assign students to perform an adult screening physical examination with supervision on a client.
- Suggest that students always do a brief head-to-toe physical examination on all clients. Have them check their findings with those described in the chart.
- Assign students to observe basic assessment skills of a nurse practitioner. If possible, allow students to perform some of the techniques during the examination.

CLINICAL CONFERENCE ACTIVITIES

- Discuss what physical assessment skills are essential for the nurse in an acute care setting, in a community setting, or in independent practice.
- Discuss how the findings during a physical examination affect the plan of care.

Critical Points to Emphasize

- The Physical examination consists of collecting objective data that is used to validate the client's subjective data (health history).
- The extent and depth of the physical examination are determined by the client's needs and the nurse's expertise.
- Physical examination is a skill used by all nurses in all settings.
- Physical examination consists of both technical skills and thinking skills. Technical skills include learning to use the equipment and correct examination techniques.
- Thinking skills include knowing *why* examination is being conducted, *how* to conduct the exam, *when* each type of exam is appropriate or indicated, and *how* to communicate the results. It also includes knowing when the data is normal or abnormal and when the data should be referred to another healthcare provider for further evaluation. In addition, the physical assessment skills are used to evaluate the effectiveness of healthcare interventions.
- The physical examination requires use of the eyes, ears, and senses of touch and smell. It takes practice to learn techniques and to use the skills.
- The physical examination requires comparing the data with standards and having a good general knowledge of anatomy (structure) and physiology (function).
- The purpose of physical examination is to differentiate normal from abnormal physical findings.
- Types of physical examination include:
  - —*Screening*: an organized superficial check of the major body systems for detecting abnormalities or possible problems.
  - —*Regional or Branching*: an in-depth assessment of a specific body system.
  - —*Comprehensive*: an in-depth assessment plus laboratory and diagnostic tests.
  - —*Periodic:* a baseline assessment to identify changes in the client's health status.
- The techniques of physical examination include inspection, palpation, percussion, and auscultation. Figure 12–1 gives an overview of these techniques.
- Guidelines for the physical examination
  - —preparation of the environment
  - —preparation of the equipment
  - —preparation of the client
    - draping
    - positioning
    - psychological preparation
  - —preparation of the examiner
  - —organization
    - sequence of examination
    - knowledge of structure and function
  - —health teaching
  - —terminating the assessment
  - —processing the information
- Points to Ponder:
  - —Measurement and recording of vital signs and other client data is often delegated to other personnel. Even though the task of collecting the data has been delegated, the nurse remains responsible for the review and interpretation of data as well as the full assessment of the client. Verification of the competency of personnel under the nurse's leadership is assumed by the agency during orientation and annually thereafter. However, nurses should develop an ongoing assessment of the skills and learning needs of the personnel under their leadership. This is especially important in today's healthcare environment where team nursing is practiced.
  - —More unlicensed workers are performing skills traditionally performed by licensed nurses.

CHAPTER

13

Diagnostic Testing

Objectives

13.1 Discuss the purpose of diagnostic testing.

13.2 Describe the various types of diagnostic testing.

13.3 Discuss the nursing responsibilities for diagnostic testing.

13.4 Discuss aspects of diagnostic testing that are commonly delegated to other personnel under the supervision of the nurse.

Facilitating Student Learning

CLASSROOM

Class Assignments

- Assign students to complete the section in the Study Guide.
- Suggest that students bring to class any questions or comments on any areas of the Study Guide that they either do not understand or need further discussion.

Lecture/Discussion

- Use the "Critical Points to Emphasize" to cover main points.
- Discuss the concepts of invasive versus noninvasive diagnostic testing.
- Give examples of invasive diagnostic tests with varying degrees of risk to the client (i.e., phlebotomy is considered minimal risk and liver biopsy is considered moderate risk)
- Discuss pre- and posttest responsibilities.

Group Activity

- Divide the class into small groups. Give each group a diagnostic test and have them teach the class. Allow five minutes per group plus about 10–15 minutes to debrief and summarize.

CLINICAL

Clinical Site Activities

- Assign students to clients undergoing some type of diagnostic test.
- Ask the students to compare and contrast their clients with a classical textbook picture.
- Assign students to a department where they do diagnostic testing to observe several types of diagnostic testing.
- Ask students to list the different types of diagnostic tests that have been ordered and have them categorize them as invasive or noninvasive.

Clinical Conference Activities

- Ask any student who has had the opportunity to observe any type of diagnostic test to share that experience. Discuss the major nursing responsibilities.
- Ask the students to share their list of diagnostic tests with the group. Lead the group in categorizing the types of tests. Discuss the similarities and differences in nursing responsibilities among the various types of tests.
- Develop a game (like *Jeopardy*) to cover the various tests and aspects of care.

Critical Points to Emphasize

- *Diagnostic testing* refers to the various methods used to assess body structure and functions.
- General Nursing Management
  - *Assess* the client's ability to participate in testing, physical condition, sensory limitations, psychological status, and functional ability.
  - *Independent nursing interventions* include client preparation, data collection, collection and transport of clients and specimens, as well as monitoring clients during and after testing.
- Refer to Box 13–1 page 56 for information on obtaining adequate specimens.
- Interdependent nursing interventions include transcribing orders, consulting with laboratory and radiology technicians, preparing the client for the test, and interpreting test results to determine if immediate action is required by the physician.
- Five "rights" of specimen collection
  - right client
  - right test
  - right specimen
  - right method of collection
  - right container
- Types of Tests
  - Microbiology Studies
  - Blood Studies
  - Urine Studies
  - Diagnostic Imaging
  - X-Ray Studies
  - Contrast X-Rays
  - Computed Tomography (CT)
  - Magnetic Resonance Imaging (MRI)
  - Positron Emission Tomography (PET)
  - Ultrasonography
  - Angiography
  - Radionuclide Scanning
  - Endoscopy
  - Cytologic Studies (nursing responsibilities include preprocedure care, intraprocedure care, and postprocedure care)

CHAPTER

14

The Cell

Objectives

14.1 Compare and contrast the general structure and function of prokaryotic and eukaryotic cells.

14.2 Discuss the structure and function of the major cell components.

14.3 Discuss the process of cell replication.

14.4 Describe alterations in cellular structure and function.

14.5 Discuss various mechanisms of cellular injury.

Facilitating Student Learning

CLASSROOM

Class Assignments

- Ask students to study the terms listed in the Study Guide.
- Assign students to review cell anatomy and physiology.

Lecture/Discussion

- Emphasize the importance of knowing normal anatomy and physiology of the cell by giving examples of application; e.g., receptors on the cell membrane determine the action of insulin, manipulation of DNA through genetic engineering to produce insulin, interferon, etc.
- Review with students the major structures and functions within the cell.
- Include the types of cells that cannot be reproduced when discussing cellular reproduction.
- Discuss the aging cell and how the immune system weakens with age.
- Provide students with common examples of client disorders that have cellular bases; e.g., myocardial infarctions cancer, cirrhosis of the liver.

CLINICAL

Clinical Site Activities

- Ask students to find actual cases of cell injury and to identify the responsible stressors.
- Ask students to find examples of the three major types of cellular alterations: 1) degeneration or infiltration, 2) genetic disturbances, 3) disorders of cell growth including malignant growth, atrophy, and hypertrophy.
- Assign students to investigate the cellular function of the medications they are administering.

Clinical Conference Activity

- Discuss students' findings in relation to cellular injury and alterations.

CHAPTER

15

Fluid and Electrolyte Disorders

Objectives

15.1 Define terms related to fluid and electrolyte imbalance.

15.2 Discuss the concepts of fluid pressures resulting in fluid movement and osmolality balance and imbalance.

15.3 Describe the etiologic factors and pathophysiology that underlie fluid volume imbalances, with and without osmolality abnormalities.

15.4 Describe the etiologic factors and pathophysiology that underlie potassium ion imbalances.

15.5 Describe the etiologic factors and pathophysiology that underlie calcium ion imbalances.

15.6 Describe the etiologic factors and pathophysiology that underlie magnesium ion imbalances.

15.7 Accurately assess a person's fluid and electrolyte status.

15.8 Identify people who are at risk for developing fluid and electrolyte imbalances and identify the specific imbalances that they are likely to incur.

15.9 Describe the nursing assessment and interventions involved in replacing fluid via the oral route and by parenteral administration.

15.10 Assess for iatrogenic complications arising from intervention in fluid and electrolyte imbalances.

15.11 Prevent fluid and electrolyte imbalance by presenting clear learning/teaching guidelines to the person and significant others.

Facilitating Student Learning

CLASSROOM

Review Activities

- Ask the students to use a book on nursing fundamentals to review the basic concepts of fluid and electrolytes.
- Ask students to review the terms related to fluid and electrolyte balance listed in the Study Guide and to learn any terms unfamiliar to them.
- Give students a nongraded pretest on the basic concepts involved in fluid and electrolyte balances and imbalances.

Class Assignments

- Assign students to complete the activities presented in the Study Guide.
- Assign students to complete the Student Worksheets for this chapter in the Study Guide.

Lecture/Discussion

- If the pretest results (see Review Activities) indicate a need, outline the basic concepts involved in fluid and electrolyte balance and imbalances. Topics to include in this presentation are body water requirements and function, the distribution and balance of body water, the chemical nature and physiologic function of electrolytes and plasma proteins, and the distribution and balance of electrolytes.
- Emphasize the importance of nurses knowing this content by listing conditions that may lead to fluid and electrolyte imbalances or by presenting a situation of a person with a condition that produced an imbalance and consequential complications. Relate how early, accurate assessment and intervention could prevent the complications. For example, an elderly gentleman has elective surgery for BPH, multiple irrigations with the TURP, and returns to the general urology unit for postop care. The afternoon of the first postop day, he is confused and a check on his a.m. serum sodium shows 124 mEq/L. Another specimen is obtained and his serum sodium is 116 mEq/L and he is having mild seizures. Since surgery he had been receiving $D_5$1/2 normal saline (NS) IV. A thorough nursing assessment that morning could have resulted in a call to the physician to change the IV fluid to NS and probably would have prevented the neurologic symptoms. Although the text lists hypertonic saline (3%) as treatment, this is rarely necessary. If hypertonic saline is given, it must be given very slowly to prevent fluid overload from a sudden increase in intravascular volume. This often results in acute pulmonary edema, pleural effusions, and cardiac tamponade. See the Case Study in the Study Guide.
- Be sure that students understand the concepts of fluid shifts between compartments and osmolality. Explain that body fluids shift between the interstitial and the intravascular spaces at the capillaries as a result of differences in hydrostatic and oncotic pressures. Explain how serum Na^+ is an indicator of fluid balance in that "water goes where salt is." Emphasize that brain cells can adapt to gradual changes in serum sodium levels but that acute changes cause cellular swelling or shrinkage with resulting neurologic signs and symptoms. Then, discuss the fluid imbalances of excess and deficit. Transparencies 4(T), 6(T), 7(T), and 8(T) may be used.
- Discuss the nurse's responsibilities in fluid replacement. Use the "Bridge to Home Care: Managing IV Therapy at Home" in the text.
- Discuss the nurse's responsibilities in the following treatments for fluid overload: fluid restriction, sodium-restricted diet, and diuretic therapy.
- Discuss nursing care for persons with specific fluid and electrolyte imbalances including assessment and interventions to prevent and treat the problem. Refer students to Tables 15–1 through 15–17 in the text for excellent summaries of important information.

- Help students understand that lab values reported in decimals cannot vary much to be within normal limits; e.g., serum K^+ of 3.5 mEq/L is normal but 2.5 mEq/L can result in cardiac arrest. On the other hand, a serum Na^+ of 135 mEq/L is normal and a value of 125 mEq/L is abnormal. Yet this low serum Na^+ may produce no symptoms or problems unless it is a sudden change. The brain can adapt to slow changes in serum Na^+ levels.

TRANSPARENCIES

- 4(T)—Pressure Differences Resulting in Fluid Shifts
- 5(T)—Chvostek's and Trousseau's Sign
- 6(T), 7(T), 8(T)—ECG Changes with Potassium Imbalance

GROUP ACTIVITIES

- Divide the class into small groups to work on case studies involving persons experiencing fluid and electrolyte imbalances. Ask each group to identify the problem, predisposing factors, appropriate nursing diagnoses and interventions (including those interventions done in collaboration with other members of the health-care team), and health teaching that may apply to prevent another occurrence.
- Using the same case studies, ask the student groups to identify the pathophysiologic basis for the signs and symptoms.

CLINICAL

SKILLS LABORATORY

- Assign students to study their clinical setting's standards of care (including policies, protocols, and procedures) pertaining to IV therapy, intake and output, and tube feedings.
- Assign students to practice the procedures of IV insertion, care of the IV site, and hanging and regulation of IV fluids. Show students various devices and equipment. They may practice IV insertion on each other using small gauge minicaths or on an IV arm mannequin using larger gauge devices.
- Demonstrate the use of an infusion pump. Stress the importance of following manufacturer's directions (for example, keeping alarm switch on while pump is in use), marking the IV bag with time and fluid levels to double check flow rate, and continuing to assess the patient and check the safe operation of the equipment.

CLINICAL SITE ACTIVITIES

- Assign students to clients with fluid and electrolyte imbalances.
- Ask students to correlate laboratory data with their assessments of a client's fluid and electrolyte status.
- Assign students to review charts to determine 1) if the charting of intravenous therapy, intake and output, tube feedings, etc., indicates that hospital policy, protocols, and procedures are being followed, 2) the incidence of complications with fluid and electrolyte therapy, and 3) if there is a correlation between 1) and 2).
- Assign individual students to work with a member of the morning "blood-drawing team" from the hospital laboratory so the students may gain experience with venipunctures.

CLINICAL CONFERENCE ACTIVITY

- Ask each student to participate in case presentations of fluid and electrolyte imbalances that have occurred in individuals assigned to them that week. Ask the students to describe their nursing assessments and correlate these with the individual's laboratory results and the nursing interventions that were used.

CHAPTER

16

Acid-Base Disorders

Objectives

16.1 Discuss general concepts of acid-base balance to include regulation and compensation to correct imbalances by the respiratory, urinary, and blood buffer systems.

16.2 Describe the etiologic factors and pathophysiology that underlie respiratory acidosis, respiratory alkalosis, metabolic acidosis, and metabolic alkalosis.

16.3 Describe in detail the nursing assessment, diagnosis, and interventions that relate to each imbalance.

Facilitating Student Learning

CLASSROOM

Review Activities

- Ask the students to use a book on physiology to review the basic concepts on acid-base balance. The textbook includes an overview of normal acid-base balance at the beginning of this chapter.
- Give students a nongraded pretest on the basic concepts involved in acid-base balance.

Class Assignment

- Assign students to complete the activities presented in the Study Guide.

Lecture/Discussion

- If the pretest results indicate a need (see Review Activities), outline the basic concepts involved in acid-base balance. Topics to include in this presentation are definition of pH, hydrolysis reaction and regulation of volatile acids by the lungs through exhalation of carbon dioxide, regulation of nonvolatile acids by the kidneys through excretion, the buffer systems, and electrolytes involved in acid-base balance.
- Emphasize the importance of nurses knowing this content by listing conditions that may lead to acid-base imbalances.
- Be sure that students understand the concept of compensation and how this differs from correction (Compensation is accomplished by the body's regulatory mechanisms and the body does not overcompensate). With compensation, the pH will be within normal limits but closer to the imbalance; e.g., if compensated acidosis, the pH will be closer to 7.35 than 7.45. Correction (accomplished by medical intervention) is best aimed at treating the underlying problem. If medication (e.g., sodium bicarbonate) is given, the pH needs to be monitored closely as overcorrection is possible, creating another acid-base imbalance.
- Discuss mixed or complex acid-base imbalances. This is particularly important in that students need to understand that the pH can be normal but the client could have severe acidosis and alkalosis. For example, respiratory acidosis can result from cardiac tamponade and metabolic alkalosis from a preexisting medical condition.
- Discuss the nurse's responsibilities in obtaining arterial blood specimens and in interpreting lab results. Table 16–2 "Sources of Error in Sampling of Arterial Blood Gases," Box 16–1 "Analysis of Arterial Blood Gases (ABGs)," and the Acid-Base Map in Figure 16–7 may be used.
- Discuss the nurse's responsibilities in the management of acid-base imbalances. The "Care Plan" section of this chapter in the text includes specific nursing diagnoses with nursing interventions and rationales appropriate for the client with acid-base imbalances.
- Discuss nursing care for clients with specific acid-base imbalances, assessment, and interventions to prevent and treat the problem. Refer students to the care plans in Figures 16–1 through 16–13 in the text.

Transparencies

- 9(T)—Regulation of Acid-Base Balance
- 10(M)—Blood Parameters of Acid-Base Imbalances

Group Activities

- Divide the class into small groups to work on case studies involving persons experiencing acid-base imbalances. Ask each group to identify the problem, predisposing factors, appropriate nursing diagnoses and interventions (including those interventions done in collaboration with other members of the healthcare team), and health teaching that may be applied to prevent another occurrence.

- Using the same case studies, ask the student groups to identify the pathophysiologic basis for the signs and symptoms (e.g., increased neuromuscular activity occurring with alkalosis is due to hypocalcemia [calcium does not ionize as well in an alkaline environment but forms a salt; therefore, the client may need supplemental calcium intravenously]).
- Provide groups of students with a list of blood gas values and ask them to identify the acid-base imbalance. Refer them to the Acid-Base Map in their text and in the Study Guide so they may check their answers. Box 16–1 "Analysis of Arterial Blood Gases (ABGs)" in the text gives them the steps to use in analyzing blood gases. The blood gas values in the Study Guide could be used or additional ones could be obtained from the lab. Transparencies 9(T) and 10(M) may be used. When using Transparency Master 10(M), remind them that CO_2 may be thought of as the CO_2 in the bicarbonate ion (HCO_3^-) and that this CO_2 is from venous blood and is one of the four main electrolytes checked routinely in a "lyte group" (NA^+, K^+, Cl^-, CO_2); whereas the pCO_2 may be thought of as acid with CO_2 combining with H_2O to form H_2CO_3.
- Another helpful hint is that the pH and pCO_2 values give the acid-base imbalance. First the student looks at the pH and decides if the imbalance is acidosis or alkalosis. Then ask the student to draw directional arrows for the pH and the pCO_2 values. If the arrows go in opposite directions, then the primary problem is respiratory; e.g., if the pH is below normal and the pCO_2 is above normal, then the primary problem is respiratory. If the arrows go the same direction, then the primary problem is metabolic; if the pH is below normal and the pCO_2 is below normal, then the primary problem is metabolic.

CLINICAL

Skills Laboratory

- Assign students to observe for an hour in a lab that runs blood gases to learn the importance of obtaining a "good specimen" (Table 16-2 "Sources of Error in Sampling of Arterial Blood Gases").
- Assign individual students to accompany a respiratory therapist to observe the procedure of drawing arterial blood specimens.

Clinical Site Activities

- Assign students to individuals with potential or actual acid-base imbalances.
- Ask students to correlate laboratory data with their assessments of an individual's acid-base status.

Clinical Conference Activity

- Ask each student to participate in case presentations of acid-base imbalances occurring in individuals assigned to them that week. Ask the students to describe their nursing assessments and correlate these with clients' laboratory results and the nursing interventions used.

Critical Points to Emphasize

Respiratory Acidosis	Respiratory Alkalosis	Metabolic Acidosis	Metabolic Alkalosis
• pH < 7.35, pCO_2 > 45 mmHg • Due to hyperventilation (e.g., with respiratory infections, chest trauma, depression of medullary respiratory center, neuromuscular diseases affecting the respiratory muscles) • Often occurs with COPD • Carbon dioxide retained • When compensated, pH normal, pCO_2 > 45 mmHg, and HCO_3 > 26 mEq/L	• pH > 7.45, pCO_2 < 35 mmHg • Due to hyperventilation (e.g., with anxiety, iatrogenically by ventilator set on high rate or large volume) • May occur with hypoxemia • Carbon dioxide exhaled • When compensated, pH normal, pCO_2 < 35 mmHg, and HCO_3 < 22 mEq/L • Too rapid correction may cause post-hypercapnic metabolic acidosis	• pH < 7.35, pCO_2 usually less than 35 mmHg, HCO_3 < 22 mEq/L • Due to acid increase or base loss • Anion gap is serum Na^+ - (Cl^- + HCO_3^-); normal = 12–14mEq/L • High anion gap occurs with acid increase; e.g., renal failure, lactic acidosis, ketoacidosis • Normal anion gap occurs with loss of base; e.g., diarrhea, enteric drainage • When compensated, pH normal, pCO_2 < 35 mmHg, HCO_3 < 22 mEq/L	• pH > 7.45, HCO_3 > 26 mEq/L • Due to acid loss (vomiting or gastric suction) or base increase (receiving $NaHCO_3$) or loss of Cl^- which causes a compensatory increase of $NaHCO_3$ • With hypovolemia or aldosterone excess, alkalosis persists (Na^+ retained and H^+ excreted) • Volume repletion with normal saline administration often corrects alkalosis if problem is not aldosterone excess

CHAPTER

17

Pain

Objectives

17.1 Discuss the multidimensional phenomenon of pain.

17.2 Discuss physiologic, psychosocial, and theoretical aspects related to the process of pain.

17.3 Discuss the types of pain and pain syndromes.

17.4 Describe the process of pain assessment.

17.5 Discuss nursing interventions for the person with pain.

17.6 Compare and contrast analgesics and various methods of analgesic administration.

17.7 Describe surgical procedures directed at relieving pain.

17.8 Describe stimulation therapies used in pain control.

Facilitating Student Learning

CLASSROOM

Review Activity

- Ask students to review material on pain in a nursing fundamentals text, such as, Bolander, V. R. (1994). *Sorenson & Luckmann's Basic Nursing: A Psychophysiologic Approach*, 3rd ed. Philadelphia: W.B. Saunders Co.

Class Assignments

- Assign students to complete the questions in the Study Guide.
- Ask students to develop a list of facilities available in the local community for the treatment of pain.
- Assign students to obtain the Agency for Healthcare Policy and Research (AHCPAR) *Guidelines on Management of Acute Pain and Management of Cancer Pain.*

Lecture/Discussion

- Discuss with students the physiologic and psychosocial aspects of pain.
- Discuss the gate-control theory of pain and use the example of biostimulation therapy (for example, transcutaneous electrical nerve stimulator [TENS]) as one approach to pain management based on this theory.
- Discuss the differences between acute, chronic, and malignant pain. Include usefulness; effect on the individual; purpose of recommended treatments regarding relief, control, or prevention; and specific differences in recommended treatments.
- Spend some time on learning experiences directed toward the affective domain to encourage students to develop empathy for people experiencing pain. The discussion of ethical issues in the text may provide assistance with this process. Ask a student from each group to share the highlights of their group discussion. (See Group Activities.)
- Using case studies of individuals experiencing different types of pain, lead a class discussion that applies the nursing process to each case and includes appropriate therapeutic approaches to pain management for each case.
- Use the AHCPAR *Guidelines on Management of Acute Pain and Cancer Pain* to discuss clinical practice in pain management.

Guest Speakers

- Invite a clinical nurse specialist or a hospice nurse who work in the area of pain management to discuss their experiences.
- Invite an anesthesiologist who works in pain management to discuss new interventions in pain management and treatment for clients with chronic pain.
- Invite a pharmacist to discuss analgesics and compare and contrast relative dosing of various agents.

Group Activities

- Divide the class into small groups to discuss personal pain experiences. Encourage them to describe when and in what circumstances the pain occurred; what they did about the pain; who they told and how; who, if anyone, was able to help; what relieved the pain; why they thought they had the pain; how they felt about the pain experience at the time; and how they feel about it now. This discussion will help students clarify beliefs about pain and suffering. It is important for student to realize how their own beliefs affect the nursing care they provide for people experiencing pain.
- Discuss with others classic "unanswerable" questions about pain such as: Why do people experience pain? Is there any purpose in suffering? What does pain mean? Consider each question from physical, emotional, and intellectual points of view. Encourage students to think about how their moral and spiritual beliefs affect their points of view.

CLINICAL

Skills Laboratory

- Assign pairs of students to practice behavioral techniques (such as meditation, relaxation, guided imagery) and physical therapies (such as massage and the application of heat and cold).
- Show students a TENS unit and a pump for self-administration of pain-relieving medications (patient-controlled analgesia [PCA]).

Clinical Site Activities

- Assign students to care for individuals experiencing pain and encourage each student to develop an individualized nursing care plan for pain management.
- Assign students to use the pain assessment tools described in the textbook.
- Ask students to audit several charts to determine if the assessment, intervention, and evaluation phases of the nursing process have been adequately recorded for nursing diagnoses associated with pain.
- Assign students to spend time in various facilities in the community for the treatment of pain to explore community options, determine what kinds of pain are treated, and determine the cost of various programs, insurance coverage, and how people gain access to the facility.

Clinical Conference Activities

- Explore with students how they view caring for individuals with various types of pain (acute versus chronic pain, pain with multiple trauma versus pain with a terminal illness, first day postoperative pain versus pain several days after surgery, pain following minor surgery versus pain following major surgery, etc.).
- Discuss the results of the chart audits (see Clinical Site Activities) and suggest improvements.
- Ask students to give case presentations of individuals experiencing pain and discuss the nursing interventions they used to help the individuals alleviate or control pain. If their evaluation indicates an intervention was not effective, ask the group what else may have worked.
- Discuss with the students the results of their use of the pain assessment tools.

CHAPTER

18

Sleep and Sensory Disorders

Objectives

18.1 Define terms associated with sleep and sensory disorders.

18.2 Discuss the physiology of sleep and arousal.

18.3 Discuss the clinical manifestations and medical management of dyssomnias.

18.4 Discuss the clinical manifestations and medical management of parasomnias.

18.5 Discuss sleep disorders associated with medical and psychiatric diseases.

18.6 Describe the impact of drugs on the sleep-wake cycle.

18.7 Discuss hospital-acquired sleep disturbances.

18.8 Describe hospital-acquired sensory disturbances.

18.9 Demonstrate appropriate nursing management of the client with a sleep disorder.

Facilitating Student Learning

CLASSROOM

Class Assignments

- Ask students to complete the section in the Study Guide before class session.
- Ask students to monitor their own sleep-wake cycle for a week. Instruct them to include time they went to bed, time they began trying to go to sleep, time of any nocturnal awakenings, time they woke in the morning, and time they actually got out of bed. Ask the students to record any naps or rest periods taken during the daytime.
- Ask students to identify factors that alter their sleep patterns. Have them indicate what factors promote rest and sleep for them.
- Assign students to interview a parent of a preschooler. Have them ask the parents to describe a typical twenty-four hour sleep pattern for the child.
- Arrange for students to visit a sleep disorder clinic or laboratory.
- Assign students to summarize an article from a nursing journal on the nursing management of a client with a sensory or sleep disorder.
- Assign students to develop drug cards for three drugs that promote rest and sleep and three drugs that interfere with rest and sleep. Instruct them to expand on the implications for the nurse.

Lecture/Discussion

- Discuss the physiology of sleep and arousal.
- If circadian rhythms have not been discussed earlier in the curriculum, you might want to include a brief overview at this point.
- Discuss factors in the hospital that interfere with rest and sleep. Ask the students to suggest sleep-promoting strategies.
- Have the class practice relaxation techniques that can be used with clients experiencing sleep disturbances.
- Discuss medical and psychiatric disorders that might contribute to sleep disturbance. Ask students to suggest appropriate nursing strategies.
- If the students were not required to develop drug cards, you will need to spend some time in class discussing sedatives and hypnotics. In addition, give examples of drugs that interfere with sleep and rest (e.g., stimulants).
- Discuss the physiologic basis of sensory/perceptual disorders.
- Help the students identify nursing diagnoses appropriate for the client with a sleep or sensory disorder.

Group Activity

- Divide the class into pairs and have the students practice collecting a sleep history.

Guest Speaker

- Invite a specialist from a sleep disorder clinic to discuss diagnostic testing and treatment of specific disorders.

CLINICAL

Clinical Site Activities

- Assign students to collect a sleep history from a young adult client and an elderly client. Ask students to compare the two histories and explain possible causes for any significant differences.
- Ask students to assess the clinical areas for factors that might contribute to sensory deprivation or overload.
- Instruct students to develop nursing diagnoses, expected outcomes, and interventions appropriate for a client with a sleep or sensory disorder.
- Arrange for students to observe an electroencephalogram.

Clinical Conference Activities

- Ask students to share their data about sensory overload or deprivation. Have the conference group suggest measures that might reduce sensory deprivation or overload in assigned clinical setting.
- Bring tracings from several sleeping electroencephalograms. Help students identify the sleep stages from the tracings. Have the students compare the tracings of different clients in the same sleep stage.

Critical Points to Emphasize

- *Sleep* can be defined as a normal state of altered consciousness during which the body rests and from which the body can be aroused by external stimuli.
- Sleep disturbances may be secondary to situational, environmental, or developmental stressors, or they may be associated with illness or with preexisting disorders.
- Sleep pattern disturbances contribute to sensory disorders, such as intensive-care psychosis.
- The sleep wake cycle is one of the circadian rhythms of the body. It follows a 24-hour pattern through a process linked to light and dark.
- Ultradian cycles are biorhythms of less than 24 hours. The recurrent patterns of sleep stages, repeating approximately every 90 minutes in adults, is an example of an ultradian cycle.
- Sleep is such an integral part of our being that it is often overlooked or minimized in the nurse's assessment and plan of care. The nurse's knowledge of the physiology of sleep, the stages of sleep , disorders of sleep, and medications that affect sleep can greatly influence the management of sleep disorders.

Selected Hospital-Acquired Sleep Disorders

PROBLEM	*CAUSE*	*IMPLICATIONS*
Sleep Onset Difficulty	• Strange environment and anxieties associated with illness and hospitalization.	• Hypnotics are often administered to hospitalized clients. Nurses should be aware of the drug's side effects.
Sleep Maintenance Disturbance	• May be associated with sustained use of or withdrawal from a variety of medications or substances. • Internal stimuli such as pain or the urge to void. • External stimuli such as lighting, noise, and temperature.	• A medication and recreational drug history is needed to identify clients at risk. • Organize nursing care and medications administration to allow for maximum periods of rest.
Sleep Deprivation	• Common disorder especially in the critical care units where the clients' conditions require frequent monitoring and nursing care.	• As above.

Selected Sleep Disorders

DISORDER	ETIOLOGY	SIGNS AND SYMPTOMS	TREATMENT
• Insomnia (Psychophysiologic insomnia is the most common insomnia.)	• Risk factors —The onset or exacerbation of illness —Hospitalization —Stress • Definition: —Learned sleep-preventing associations and heightened physiologic responses to stress.	• Inability to sleep or maintain sleep • Frequent awakenings • Excessive daytime sleepiness	• Difficult to treat • Referral to a sleep specialist or mental health professional who can work with client over a period of time should be considered.
• Narcolepsy (Characterized by excessive daytime sleepiness. Safety is major issue. Sixty to eighty percent of clients with narcolepsy report falling asleep at work and while driving.)	• The cause of narcolepsy is thought to be linked to a malfunctioning of the mechanism controlling REM sleep. • Narcolepsy is a genetically heterogeneous condition with a prevalence of 1 in 1000 persons in the United States.	• Irresistible daytime drowsiness followed by brief periods of sleep, especially when engaged in monotonous activities. • Cataplexy—sudden loss of muscle tone at unexpected times. • Sleep paralysis—The inability to move upon initial awakening.	• Diagnosis is by history and polysomnography. • Medical management consists of low doses of stimulants to improve alertness and tricyclic antidepressants to control cataplexy. • Stress the importance of maintaining a regular sleep schedule. • Regular naps at the times clients are prone to sleepiness may be helpful.

(Continued)

Selected Sleep Disorders

(Concluded)

DISORDER	ETIOLOGY	SIGNS AND SYMPTOMS	TREATMENT
• Sleep Apnea Syndrome—Obstructive Sleep Apnea (OSAS). (Affects 1% of adult population. Increased incidence in middle-aged males and certain occupations such as truck driving. Clients that snore, are obese, and/or have short, thick necks are at risk for sleep apnea.)	• Exact cause is unknown. • Respiratory efforts of the diaphragm and intercostal muscles are apparent but ineffective against a collapsed or obstructed upper airway.	• Hypnagogic hallucinations—hallucinatory experiences that occur at sleep onset or awakening. • Escalating snoring followed by a silent pause, which ends with a gasp or snort. • Hypoxia • Frequent awakenings • Excessive daytime sleepiness	• Mild cases —Weight reduction —Sleep in positions other than supine • Severe Cases —CPAP (continuous positive airway pressure) —Uvulopalatopharyngoplasty (UPPP) —Tracheostomy —Oral and dental appliances may help to maintain a patent airway —Refer to Client Education Guide in text: Living with OSAS • Referral to sleep disorders center for clients observed to have repeated periods of apnea (one a minute, or more than 15 to 20 periods an hour) lasting longer that 10 seconds, with or without snoring.

CHAPTER

19

Infectious Disorders

OBJECTIVES

19.1 Discuss factors involved in the transmission and development of infectious disease.

19.2 Obtain a nursing history that will help to identify the person at risk for developing an infectious disease.

19.3 Perform specific preventive nursing measures in the healthcare setting to decrease the incidence of nosocomial infections.

19.4 Discuss universal precautions and the two tiers of isolation strategies: standard precautions and transmission-based precautions.

19.5 Discuss Occupational Safety and Health Administration (OSHA) guidelines for protecting healthcare workers exposed to blood and other potentially infectious materials.

19.6 Discuss OSHA guidelines for preventing the spread of tuberculosis in hospitals.

19.7 List recommendations for adult immunizations.

Facilitating Student Learning

CLASSROOM

Review Activity

- Ask students to review terminology related to the basic concept of infection. They may use their fundamentals of nursing text.

Class Assignments

- Assign students to study the unit or chapters on anti-infectives in their pharmacology text. Ask them to bring to class major classification drug cards which outline the modes of action, routes of administration, usual side effects, major toxic effects, nursing implications, client education, and approximate cost.
- Assign students to complete the activities in the Study Guide for Chapter 19.

Lecture/Discussion

- Give students the most recent information from Centers for Disease Control (CDC) and OSHA on infection risk, prevention, and control strategies in acute care facilities.
- Discuss the increased cost of healthcare, including prolonged hospitalization, for the client who develops an infection. Present an example of an actual case of a client who develops an infection after being admitted to a healthcare facility.
- Discuss the nurse's role in controlling the transmission of infection.
- Use laboratory reports to discuss the changes in values that occur with infection.
- Discuss the major classifications of anti-infective drugs. Emphasize nursing implications and client education.
- Discuss, in general terms, the pathophysiology of septic shock and the medical and nursing interventions for the client in septic shock. Emphasize the importance of nursing assessment of the client in septic shock. (This topic and the activity "Septic Shock" may be found in Chapter 22 of the Study Guide.)

Guest Speaker

- Invite an infection control nurse or a hospital epidemiologist to discuss aspects of infection control and an environmental safety control officer to discuss safe disposal of contaminated waste.

CLINICAL

Skills Laboratory

- Assign pairs of students to role play how they would teach wound care and dressing changes.

Clinical Site Activities

- As students administer anti-infectives, ask them to give the specific rationale for the drug's use for the client receiving the medication.
- Assign students to identify factors in the clinical setting that increase the risk of nosocomial infections, antibiotic-resistant strains of organisms, and allergic hypersensitivity of clients to antibiotics.
- Ask students to correlate signs and symptoms of infection with laboratory data.

Clinical Conference Activities

- Discuss the factors that the students identified in the clinical setting that increase the risk of nosocomial infections, antibiotic-resistant strains of organisms, and allergic hypersensitivity of clients to antibiotics. Discuss ways nurses can reduce the risks.
- List the anti-infective drugs the students administered. Discuss any side effects experienced by the clients receiving the medications and any precautions taken to reduce the incidence of toxic effects. Also, discuss the beneficial effects of the drug therapy.
- Discuss organization of nursing activities when providing care for clients on isolation.

CHAPTER

20

Wound Healing

Objectives

20.1 Describe the processes involved in the phases of normal wound healing.

20.2 Describe the types of wound healing intention.

20.3 Discuss the functions of various nutrients needed in wound healing.

20.4 Describe management of the client with an inflammation, incision, chronic inflammation, and open wound.

20.5 Discuss nursing management for the client with a wound.

Facilitating Student Learning

CLASSROOM

Review Activity

- Ask the students to use a nursing fundamentals text to review (a) interventions for wound care, (b) principles of sterile technique, and (c) principles of medical asepsis.

Class Assignment

- Assign students to complete the Study Guide questions for Chapter 20.

Lecture/Discussion

- Review with the students the processes involved in the four phases of wound healing.
- Refer students to Table 20–3 of the textbook, as well as readings for a class discussion on changes in laboratory values with inflammations/infections and how to interpret these changes. Use laboratory reports to discuss the changes in values that occur with inflammation and/or infection.
- Discuss the differences between acute and chronic inflammatory reactions.
- Discuss the local and systemic manifestations of inflammation. Emphasize the importance of early assessment.
- Show slides that depict various types of wound repair and healing. Use the assessment factors listed in Box 20–1 in the textbook.
- Summarize important points about wound assessment and promoting wound healing.
- Prepare a demonstration for students that includes types of dressings and indications for use.
- Discuss various agents used in treatment of open wounds, indications for use, and impact on wound healing.
- Introduce students to the American Healthcare Policy and Research (AHCPAR) guidelines for treatment of pressure sores.

Guest Speakers

- Invite a member of the nutrition support team, a nutritionist, or an enterostomal therapist to discuss the importance of nutrition in wound healing.

CLINICAL

Skills Laboratory

- Ask students to discuss in their own words the principles and process of wound healing.
- Assign students to demonstrate various nursing interventions in which they would apply the principles they have discussed. Nursing interventions may include application of heat or cold, elevation of body part, dressing change using aseptic technique, and wet to dry dressing.

Clinical Site Activities

- Assign students to care for persons with wounds at different stages in the healing process.
- Ask students to describe the wound according to 1) type of wound, 2) size of wound, 3) condition of the surrounding tissues, 4) presence of pain, 5) presence of exudates and drainage, and 6) presence of complications.
- Ask students to determine factors (internal and external) affecting wound healing in each person for whom they are providing care.
- Assign students to prepare a teaching plan for wound care for a client being discharged from the hospital.
- Arrange for students to spend some clinical time with an enterostomal therapist to assist with complex dressing changes and to assess wounds.
- Ask students to interpret laboratory reports that apply to inflammation.

Clinical Conference Activities

- Ask the students to identify the common factors affecting wound healing in persons for whom they have been providing care, and discuss the therapies and nursing diagnoses and interventions used. From this information, develop a standardized care plan for a person with a local inflammatory reaction. Also, discuss how this standardized care plan would need to be individualized for each person the students were assigned to that week.
- Assign students to bring a copy of the portion of the progress notes where they describe the wound and wound care. Ask students to record the same information on a flow sheet. Discuss the advantages of each method of charting.
- Work with students to prepare a teaching plan for wound care for a client being discharged from the hospital.

CHAPTER

21

Perioperative Nursing

Objectives

21.1 Discuss basic concepts related to perioperative nursing.

21.2 Interview a person who is to undergo surgery, gathering subjective and objective data.

21.3 Discuss the legal aspects of informed consent.

21.4 Discuss the physical, psychosocial, and teaching aspects of preoperative care.

21.5 Describe the roles of healthcare providers who participate in the intraoperative experience.

21.6 Discuss the implications of the types of anesthesia used in the operating room.

21.7 Discuss the nurse's roles in caring for the client in the operating room.

21.8 Describe nursing care of the client in the postanesthesia recovery room.

21.9 Identify elements of client assessment essential upon transfer to the nursing unit after surgery.

21.10 Discuss goals of care during the postoperative phase.

Facilitating Student Learning

CLASSROOM

Review Activities

- Review principles of teaching/learning in fundamentals text such as Bolander, V. R. (1994). *Sorensen & Luckmann's Basic Nursing: A Psychophysiologic Approach*, 3rd ed. Philadelphia, W. B. Saunders Co.
- Review principles of asepsis for a safe intraoperative experience.

Lecture/Discussion

- Discuss physiologic factors from the history and physical that need special emphasis with the surgical client.
- Elaborate on the state laws regarding "informed consent" and local hospital policies for obtaining written and verbal consent.
- Emphasize nursing research that supports the value of preoperative teaching. (See bibliography for specific citations.)
- Discuss with students the implications for preoperative teaching of outpatient surgery, one-day surgery, and admission to the hospital the morning of surgery.
- Develop with students a preoperative teaching checklist and discuss individual teaching items.
- Emphasize to students the importance of maintaining good communication between the nurse and physician so that consistent information is given to the person having surgery.
- Share a preoperative checklist with students. Discuss the importance of early preoperative checklist preparation in light of the "fluid" nature of operating room schedules.
- Emphasize the essentials of safe nursing care for the client's intraoperative experience.
- Discuss the roles of healthcare providers in the operating room.
- Discuss the implications of agents used for general and regional anesthesia.
- Emphasize the critical elements to be assessed in the postanesthesia recovery period, upon admission to the nursing unit, and during postoperative recovery.
- Discuss nursing responsibilities in assessing, preventing, and/or treating postoperative complications.
- Discuss the elements of postoperative pain and nursing responsibilities in preventing and/or treating persons with pain.
- Discuss elements of discharge teaching.

Transparencies

- 11(T)—Types of Anesthesia
- 12(T)—Five Surgical Positions
- 13(M)—Endotracheal Tube Placement

Guest Speakers

- Invite an OR nurse to discuss nursing responsibilities for care of the client during the intraoperative phase.
- Invite a nurse anesthetist to discuss general and regional anesthetics and their implications.

CLINICAL

Skills Laboratory

- Assign students to demonstrate teaching coughing, deep breathing, incentive spirometry, turning, and leg exercises to the client having surgery.
- Assign students to practice positioning each other in the various surgical positions.

Clinical Site Activities

- Assign students to persons scheduled for surgery. Have students complete a preoperative interview and estimate the person's surgical risk.
- Assign student to preoperative clients. Have students do the admission assessment, preoperative teaching, skin and GI preparation, preoperative checklist, and medications.

- Assign students to accompany clients to the OR. Have students identify learning objectives for the experience. Some suggested areas could include safety, care of the unconscious person, principles of asepsis, and roles of the surgical team members.
- Assign students to accompany their OR clients to the recovery room or assign them to the recovery room for a day. As part of their assignment, ask students to write up their initial baseline assessment of one person, participate in receiving the verbal report from the OR team, assist the recovery room nurses with safe positioning and nursing care, and write up their ongoing assessment of the client recovering from anesthesia.
- Assign students in their recovery room experience to review the anesthesia record for the types of anesthesia used and identify the implications for nursing assessment and care.
- Assign students to clients returning to the nursing unit from the recovery room. Assist them to identify equipment to have on hand and baseline assessments they will need to make on the client.
- Using the goals for postoperative care from the text, assign students to develop a nursing care plan for a postoperative client.
- Assign students to plan and implement discharge planning for a person who has had surgery.

Clinical Conference Activities

- Ask students to discuss and compare preoperative client preparation experiences focusing on the information needs of clients and their significant others. Discuss with students the quote by Sir Berkley Mynehan, "For us an operation is an incident in a day's work, but for our patient it may be, and no doubt often is, the sternest and most dreadful of all trials, for the mysteries of life and death surround it, and it must be faced alone."
- Focus student discussions of their OR experience to include functions of the circulating nurse, safety (environmental and client), and surgical positioning.
- Based on the various surgeries that the students observed, lead a student discussion on physiological reasons that persons having surgery have pain postoperatively.
- Assign different students to present one of the potential postoperative complications from the recovery room period, upon immediate return to the nursing unit, or during recovery. Have students discuss how to assess for the complications and how to prevent or treat them if they occur.
- Invite a respiratory therapist to postconference to discuss principles of and demonstrate techniques used with incentive spirometry devices and to discuss rationale for using incentive spirometry.

CHAPTER

22

Shock

Objectives

22.1 Discuss basic etiologies of shock.

22.2 Identify similarities and differences among various types of shock.

22.3 Describe generally recognized stages of shock and possible consequences of each.

22.4 Explain the systemic effects of shock.

22.5 Recognize the early assessment findings indicating shock.

22.6 List potential nursing diagnoses for the client in shock.

22.7 Implement appropriate interventions for people in shock.

Facilitating Student Learning

CLASSROOM

Review Activities

- Ask students to review the circulatory system's structure and function.
- Assign students to review "Administration of Blood and Blood Products" in a fundamentals of nursing textbook.

Class Assignment

- Assign students to complete the activities for this chapter in the Study Guide.

Lecture/Discussion

- When discussing the various types of shock, help students identify similarities and see that the end results of every type of shock are the same. Transparency 209(M) may be used.
- When explaining the pathophysiologic effects of shock, emphasize that shock affects all organs because all cells in the body become hypoxic as the stages of shock progress.
- Stress the importance of early recognition of the first signs of shock in the early stages to prevent complications of shock. Emphasize checking for postural hypotension or an increase in pulse rate with a change from lying to sitting position. Transparency 211(M) may be used.
- Discuss first aid for the person in shock. Transparencies 211(M) and 212(T) may be used when discussing positioning for the person in shock and using the antishock (MAST) suit.
- Discuss the general principles and rationale for invasive and noninvasive shock assessment techniques. Transparency 213(T) may be used.
- Using a case presentation of a person in hypovolemic (hemorrhagic) shock, review assessment and first-aid intervention, and discuss definitive medical and nursing interventions.

Transparencies

- 209(M)—Types of Shock
- 210(T)—Signs and Symptoms of Shock
- 211(M)—Orthostatic Vital Signs and Positioning of Person in Shock
- 212(T)—MAST Suit
- 213(T)—Swan-Ganz Catheter

Group Activity

- Ask small groups of students to list conditions that would be more likely to predispose people to developing shock, and to categorize those conditions under the type of shock each condition is most likely to produce. With the whole class, compare lists. This activity will help students identify people at risk for developing shock.

CLINICAL

Skills Laboratory

- Assign students to review the policies and procedures pertaining to intravenous fluid and blood administration. Usually, outdated blood and blood products can be borrowed from the blood bank to make this experience more realistic.
- Ask pairs of students to demonstrate assessment and first-aid interventions for a person experiencing signs and symptoms of hemorrhagic shock.
- Demonstrate assessment of fluid status using central venous pressure monitoring. Stress the importance of a change in the individual's readings rather than the normal range of CVP values.
- Invite a nurse from the emergency department to demonstrate the use of the MAST suit.

Clinical Site Activities

- Assign students to the emergency department and trauma or critical care units to observe the care given for a person in shock if it is not feasible to assign students to assist with providing that care. Ask the students to seek information concerning the individual's total care and not to focus solely on the equipment.
- Ask students to obtain information about medications used to treat shock. The information should include the generic and trade names of the medication, usual dosage, mode of action, possible side effects, and nursing implications for administration.
- Conduct "walking rounds" on a general hospital unit with the students to help them identify persons at risk for developing shock. Ask the students how they would assess each patient for signs and symptoms of shock and how they would intervene to prevent complications.

Clinical Conference Activities

- Ask any student who has had the opportunity to work with an individual in shock to share that experience. Discuss the psychosocial assistance that was given to significant others as well as to the person being treated for shock.
- Discuss the information gathered by the students on medications to treat shock.

Critical Points to Emphasize

- *Types and Etiology*: Hypovolemic (hemorrhage, burns, dehydration); cardiogenic (myocardial infarction, pulmonary embolus); distributive (anaphylactic—acute allergic reaction; neurogenic—acute phase of spinal cord injury; septic—severe infection with sepsis).
- *Pathophysiology*: Early compensatory state (with decreased perfusion, sympathetic nervous system is stimulated and blood flow is redistributed to brain and heart); decompensation stage (decreased cardiac output with continued vasoconstriction, decreased tissue perfusion, anaerobic metabolism and lactic acidosis, dilation of microcirculation); progressive stage (cellular ischemia and necrosis, organ failure).
- *Clinical Manifestations*: Early compensatory state (normal blood pressure then narrowing of pulse pressure, tachycardia, restlessness, agitation, confusion, decreased urine output to less than 20 cc/hr, tachypnea); decompensation to progressive stage (severely low blood pressure, weak and thready pulse, dysrhythmias, lethargy, stupor, coma, decreasing urine specific gravity, anuria). Skin and mucous membranes may be flushed, warm, and moist in early septic shock; cool, pale, and moist in progressive shock; flushed with macular or papular lesions in anaphylactic shock. (See Figure 22–7 in the text for a graphic illustration.)
- *Management*: Maintain perfusion with titrating vasoconstrictors and vasodilators (see Table 22–2 in the text); improve oxygenation with oxygen and mechanical ventilation with positive-end-expiratory pressure (PEEP) if needed; assist circulation with MAST garment, intra-aortic balloon pump (IABP), modified Trendelenburg's position; replace fluid volume with colloids, blood, and crystalloids as needed; prevent renal failure by maintaining urine output greater than 40 cc/hr; prevent gastrointestinal bleeding by using gastric suction, antacids, and histamine blockers. (See Tables 22–3, 22–4, and 22–5 in the text for more specifics.)
- It is critical to recognize shock in the early compensatory stage and treat early to prevent decompensation and progressive stage of shock which has been called appropriately *irreversible shock* and leads to multiple organ failure.

CHAPTER

23

Basic Concepts of Neoplastic Disorders

OBJECTIVES

23.1 Discuss basic concepts related to cancer.

23.2 Discuss factors predisposing a person to cancer and the impact of cancer.

23.3 Compare and contrast characteristics of normal cells and cancer cells.

23.4 Discuss the nurse's role in cancer prevention and screening.

23.5 Discuss general and specific techniques involved in cancer diagnosis and the nurse's role.

Facilitating Student Learning

CLASSROOM

Review Activity

- Ask students to review Chapter 14, "The Cell," in the textbook for normal cell anatomy and physiology.

Class Assignment

- Assign students to learn the definitions of the terms listed in the Study Guide.

Lecture/Discussion

- Lead a class discussion on the topic of known and suspected cancer determinants (etiologic and predisposing factors) to identify ways to eliminate or control these factors.
- Discuss the effect of cancer on the person, significant others, and society. Include the emotional response to cancer; and the social roles of the acutely and chronically ill individual, of the individual who is dying, and of the significant others who are given the responsibilities of providing care for the individual with cancer. Also include the financial effect of cancer on the individual and significant others, as well as on the national economy.
- Emphasize the progress that has been made in cancer research in the areas of prevention, diagnosis, and treatment.
- Emphasize the role of the nurse in cancer prevention. Suggest ways that students can teach clients in their daily care; for example, by recommending to female clients over 35 to request a mammogram and pap smear while they are in the hospital or clinic.
- Assign students to visit the local chapter of the American Cancer Society to obtain information on the available educational materials on cancer prevention.
- Review the characteristics of normal cells to help students understand the changes that occur in neoplastic cells. Compare normal cell characteristics with cancer cell characteristics.
- Discuss the growth and spread of cancer cells.
- Refer students to Table 23–5 in the textbook. Help them learn to differentiate between benign and malignant neoplasms by identifying the key words for malignant neoplasms with the tissue of origin; i.e., sarcoma (connective tissue), carcinoma (epithelium), lymphoma (lymphoid tissue).
- Discuss the nurse's role in the general and specific techniques used in cancer diagnosis. Emphasize support of the client and significant others and teaching aspects.
- Discuss cancer prevention at primary, secondary, and tertiary levels.
- Describe appropriate assessment for each of the seven warning signals of cancer.

Transparencies

- 14(T)—The Cell Cycle
- 15(M)—Cancer's Seven Warning Signals

Group Activity

- Ask groups of students to list factors in their lives that are known or suspected cancer determinants and to suggest ways to eliminate or control these factors. Ask students within small groups to share their personal experiences with cancer.

Guest Speakers

- Invite a representative from the local chapter of the American Cancer Society (ACS) to discuss available educational materials on cancer prevention and services provided by the ACS to persons with cancer and significant others. Have the representative also discuss opportunities for nurses within ACS.
- Invite a member of the local chapter of the Oncology Nursing Society to discuss the nurse's role in cancer prevention.

CLINICAL

Skills Laboratory

- If a Cancer Teaching Center Laboratory is available, assign students to complete all the modules on cancer prevention; e.g., breast self-exam, testicular self-exam, smoking and smokeless tobacco use, differentiation of benign and malignant skin lesions, colorectal tests.
- Assign students to learn breast self-exam and testicular self-exam on models and to practice at home as appropriate. Encourage them to instruct others in the technique.
- Assign pairs of students to perform oral exams on each other.

Clinical Site Activities

- Assign students to a setting where they can be with persons who are having diagnostic studies for cancer detection. Ambulatory care clinics, physicians' offices, the hospital one-day surgery unit, and medical-surgical units should provide ample opportunities.
- Assign students to guaiac their client's stools. Assign students to look up the preparation for the procedure.
- In cooperation with community health nursing faculty, assign groups of students to identify a public education need related to cancer prevention in a specified community and to plan and implement a project designed to meet that identified need. One potential community facility is senior citizen residential facilities.
- As appropriate, assign students to do cancer prevention/early detection teaching with their clients.

Clinical Conference Activities

- Lead a discussion of the students' experiences with persons having diagnostic studies for cancer detection. Ask students to outline the required nursing care pre- and postdiagnostic test.
- Have students share their cancer prevention and early detection teaching projects with the group. Identify other at-risk groups where nurses and students nurses could share prevention information.

CHAPTER

24

Treatment Modalities for Neoplastic Disorders

Objectives

24.1 Discuss psychosocial aspects of the four phases of the cancer continuum.

24.2 Discuss the role of surgery in cancer treatment and diagnosis.

24.3 Discuss radiation therapy as a treatment modality for neoplastic disorders, its potential side effects, and nursing care.

24.4 Discuss chemotherapy as a treatment modality for neoplastic disorders, its side effects, and nursing care.

24.5 Discuss bone marrow transplantation and biologic response modifiers used as cancer treatment modalities.

Facilitating Student Learning

CLASSROOM

Review Activity

- Suggest students review Chapter 21 in the textbook for basic principles of preoperative and postoperative care as these apply to persons undergoing surgery for cancer.

Class Assignments

- Assign students to complete the section in the Study Guide for this chapter.
- Assign students to visit the local chapter of the American Cancer Society to obtain information on the resources available to nurses to use in continuing education and for their clients with cancer.
- Assign students to read recent issues of *Cancer Nursing: An International Journal for Cancer Care* or *Oncology Nursing Forum.* Have students share summaries of pertinent articles.
- Ask students to use their pharmacology text to review medications used in the treatment of neoplastic disorders; e.g., antineoplastic, analgesic, and antiemetic medications.

Lecture/Discussion

- Outline the important points in each treatment modality with emphasis placed on the nursing diagnoses and appropriate interventions for each.
- Assign small groups of students to investigate one of the side effects of chemotherapy or radiation therapy for the latest medical and nursing treatments. Provide students with blank transparencies to report their findings to the class.
- Discuss the unique problems of the person facing cancer surgery. Emphasize the importance of providing psychosocial support for the person and significant others.
- Lead the class discussion in developing a nursing care plan for a person in each phase of cancer therapy; e.g., diagnosis and treatment, survivorship, recurrent disease and palliation, and terminal. Clinical examples will facilitate the discussion.
- Discuss various aspects of cancer research.
- Discuss safety issues related to radiation and chemotherapy administration that affect the nurse.

Transparencies

- 16(T)—Radiation Safety
- 17(T)—Classifications of Chemotherapy
- 19(M)—Venous Access Devices
- 18(T)—Cerebrospinal Fluid Reservoir
- 20(M)—Toxic Effects of Chemotherapy

Guest Speakers

- Invite a representative from the local chapter of the American Cancer Society (ACS) to discuss the educational materials available for nurses, clients, and their families.
- Invite members of various support groups for persons with different types of cancer (e.g., Lost Chord Club, Ostomy Association, Reach to Recovery) to discuss the role of the support group in helping others with cancer and to share what nursing interventions were most helpful to them as well as suggest other interventions that would be helpful. For large classes, this strategy may work better as a clinical conference activity.
- Invite an advanced practice nurse specializing in oncology to discuss his or her role and future directions in oncology nursing.
- Invite a hospice nurse to discuss hospice philosophy and care of clients in a hospice program.
- Invite a clinical pharmacist to discuss use of antiemetics with nausea and vomiting related to chemotherapy.

Group Activities

- Give small groups of students ethical issues that they will find in working with clients with cancer. Box 24–13 in the textbook provides a list of important ethical issues. Encourage students to discuss and debate the various aspects of these issues.
- Assign each group to do a literature review of one aspect of nutrition for the person with cancer and to give a summary either in class or in clinical conference. Possible topics are control of nausea and vomiting during chemotherapy; oral care of the person with stomatitis and mucositis related to chemotherapy and radiation therapy; diet education for the person and significant others when anorexia is present related to the treatment of cancer, the psychosocial impact of cancer, and the pathophysiology of cancer.

CLINICAL

Skills Laboratory

- Demonstrate infusion devices used in the administration of chemotherapy.

Clinical Site Activities

- Assign students to provide nursing care for persons with cancer who are undergoing various treatment methods in the hospital and ambulatory care clinics.
- With the cooperation of the community health nursing faculty, assign students to follow persons with cancer from the hospital to their homes. The students could make home visits as necessary and go to the clinic with the clients. This approach helps the students learn the importance of continuity of care, discharge planning, and the role of the nurse in the community-based setting.
- Provide students with the opportunity to tour a radiation therapy facility and ask them to develop a nursing care plan for a patient receiving radiation therapy.
- Assign each student to find the healthcare facility protocol for the administration of a specific chemotherapeutic agent.
- Assign students to investigate protocols for treatment of extravasation.
- Provide students with the opportunity to attend a tumor board conference.
- Arrange for one or two interested students to attend an "I Can Cope" meeting.

Clinical Conference Activities

- Ask students to share their findings regarding the specific protocols for the administration of the various chemotherapeutic agents. Ask the class to list general nursing considerations for the administration of chemotherapeutic agents.
- Assign students to use a case presentation format to share with the group their clinical experiences with persons with cancer and to lead a class discussion for the purpose of strengthening their nursing care plan.
- Encourage students to discuss their feelings about cancer and caring for persons who have cancer.
- Invite a representative of the "Can Surmount" program to discuss their volunteer efforts to help all people with cancer.
- Ask the students who attended the "I Can Cope" meetings to share their experiences with the class.
- Focus a postconference on developing a nursing care plan for a client receiving chemotherapy with nausea and vomiting.

CHAPTER

25

Structure and Function of the Immune System

Objectives

25.1 Differentiate between active and passive immunity.

25.2 Compare and contrast humoral and cellular immunity.

25.3 Identify the organs of the immune system.

25.4 Describe the relationship of B lymphocytes and T lymphocytes, Class I and II MHC molecules, and CD4 and CD8 surface markers.

25.5 Distinguish between features of primary and secondary immune responses.

25.6 Discuss, in general terms, the characteristics of immunoglobulins (antibodies).

25.7 Describe the functions of the four types of T lymphocytes.

25.8 Describe the roles of the cytokines.

25.9 Identify the factors that affect the immune response.

Facilitating Student Learning

CLASSROOM

Class Assignment

- Assign students to complete the activities in the Study Guide for Chapter 25.

Lecture/Discussion

- Give students a brief review of the immune system. Transparencies 21(T) and 23(T) may be used. Use slides made from electron microscopy photography to show the immune system in action; i.e., a T-cell destroying a cancer cell.
- Discuss how aging affects the immune system and how the resulting decline in immune system function results in many of the diseases occurring more frequently in the elderly population.
- Discuss recent advances in immunology and the implications for nursing.

Transparencies

- 21(T)—Organs of the Immune System
- 22(T)—Components of Nonspecific Defense Mechanisms
- 23(T)—Overview of Defense Mechanisms

CLINICAL

Clinical Site Activity

- Ask students to identify factors that affect the immune response in the individuals for whom the students are providing care.

Clinical Conference Activity

- Discuss factors affecting the immune response that the students have identified while at the clinical site.

CHAPTER

26

Assessment of Clients with Immune Disorders

Objectives

26.1 Obtain a health history to determine possible allergies, including food, medication, insect, or pollen sensitivities.

26.2 Review the client's health history to identify previous problems and signs/symptoms of immune system dysfunction.

26.3 Perform a physical examination of the client and focus on the area that is target for the allergen or other immune system problem.

26.4 Describe the following diagnostic tests for AIDS: ELISA, Western Blot, and RIPA.

26.5 Differentiate among the following tests: CD4 cell counts, lymphocyte and immunoglobulin assays, lymphangiography, and skin testing. Provide a brief description of the tests, and pre- and postprocedure care if applicable.

Facilitating Student Learning

CLASSROOM

Class Assignment

- Assign students to complete the activities in the Study Guide for this chapter.

Lecture/Discussion

- Role play obtaining a medical history related to immune disorders.
- Discuss screening/diagnostic tests for AIDS, the reason for screening with ELISA and confirmatory testing with the Western Blot, the importance of maintaining confidentiality, and appropriate ways of informing the client of results.
- Discuss administration and interpretation of skin tests for allergies.

CLINICAL

Clinical Site Activities

- Assign students to an allergy clinic for a morning or day.
- Assist students with interpreting results of laboratory tests to detect problems with the immune system.

CHAPTER

27

Nursing Care of Clients with Altered Immune Systems

OBJECTIVES

27.1 Describe the following characteristics of HIV infection: definition, incidence, etiology, risk factors.
27.2 Discuss the pathophysiology and resulting clinical manifestation of HIV infection.
27.3 Identify various pharmacologic agents used in treating clients with HIV infection.
27.4 Describe the various opportunistic infections according to causative agent, symptomatology, and treatment.
27.5 List HIV-associated malignancies.
27.6 Describe central and peripheral HIV neurologic disease.
27.7 Discuss nursing care for the client with HIV infection.
27.8 Describe universal precautions.
27.9 Describe the four types of hypersensitivity reactions.
27.10 Describe self-care for the client with allergies.
27.11 Discuss the basic concepts of histocompatibility and the immunologic aspects of transplant rejection.
27.12 Describe the signs and symptoms of graft rejection and graft-versus-host disease.
27.13 Identify the basic criteria for transplantation.
27.14 Discuss nursing care for the client having a transplant.
27.15 Identify major medications used in immunosuppression.
27.16 Discuss ethical considerations associated with transplantation.

Facilitating Student Learning

CLASSROOM

Class Assignments

- Assign students to complete the activities in the Study Guide.
- Ask students to read current professional and lay literature on HIV infection.

Lecture/Discussion

- Using a case history of a client with AIDS, discuss assessment of immunodeficiency by nursing history and physical exam, appropriate laboratory diagnostic tests, classification and staging categories, medical treatment, and nursing care. Give special attention to learning/teaching for the client and significant others (include mode and prevention of transmission, signs and symptoms of infection, safe sex, handwashing, general disinfectant techniques, health maintenance, and where to seek reliable information). Refer students to the text for the listing of organizations to contact for additional information on AIDS.
- Discuss recent advances in immunology and the implications for nursing. The June 28, 1996 issue of *Science* (Volume 272, Number 5270) includes a special report on AIDS (pp. 1841-2012). Nine easy-to-read articles contain the latest information on research, pathogenesis, and treatment.

Guest Speakers

- Invite an allergist or a nurse practitioner working with people with allergies to discuss the application of new research findings in the diagnosis and treatment of allergies.
- Invite an immunologist or a clinical nurse specialist knowledgeable in that area to discuss the recent advances in immunology and its applications for diagnosis and treatment.

Group Activity

- Assign groups of students to identify appropriate items to include in a teaching plan for individuals with immunosuppression. Then use these items during a class discussion to develop a teaching plan.

CLINICAL

Clinical Site Activities

- Ask students to identify factors that affect the immune response in the individuals for whom the students are providing care.
- Assign students to an allergy clinic for a morning or day. Ask students to develop teaching plans for people receiving desensitization.
- Assist students with interpreting results of laboratory tests to detect problems with the immune system.

Clinical Conference Activities

- Discuss factors affecting the immune response that the students have identified while at the clinical site, and specific interventions used for individuals with the resulting altered immune responses. Ask the group of students if other interventions should have been included.
- Discuss the psychosocial, ethical, and legal aspects of HIV infection. Encourage the students to express their attitudes. Emphasize how clients with AIDS need nursing care, and how students can provide that care without fear of contracting the disease.
- Ask students to compare their teaching plans for persons receiving desensitization.
- Discuss the ethical issue "Do Transplant Clients Have an Obligation to Comply with Their Post-Transplant Self-Care?" outlined in the ethical issue box in the text. Ask students if they have encountered this situation with their clients and, if so, how they feel about it. Then discuss appropriate techniques to use in dealing with the situation.

Baseline Information for Long-Term Care Planning in HIV Disease

Database	Information
1. Demographics	a. Personal data—name, age, date of birth, social security number, race/ethnicity, telephone number(s), address, and life-partner b. Occupation/profession and education—job title and highest level of education c. Languages spoken—how many and which is preferred communication language d. Risk behavior for HIV infection—sex, needle exposure, blood products
2. Support person(s)	a. Living with client—who lives in the client's home b. Designated care-partner—who will assist the client when needed c. Willing to participate in plan of care—are these individuals willing to provide direct care or only available for emotional support and financial/legal matters d. Family members—where do family members (parents, siblings) live, and are they aware of diagnosis
3. Functional status	a. Physical impairments—what are the physical limitations of the client b. Mental impairments—what are the mental impairments of the client c. Activities of daily living (ADL)—are there any that the client cannot perform
4. Clinical needs	a. Medical diagnoses—all pre-existing and current medical diagnoses b. Medications ordered—current medicines ordered as well as over-the-counter medications taken routinely c. Clinical trials—is the client enrolled in a clinical trial or interested in participating d. Nutrition—patterns e. Rehabilitation needs—any therapy needs

(Continued)

Clinical needs—*con't*	f. Treatments—any routine treatments required g. Equipment/supplies—any routinely needed supplies to perform treatments h. Medical follow-up—what arrangements exist for health care follow-up i. Addiction treatment—has the client ever received treatment, currently in treatment, or interested in treatment (both alcohol and drugs)
5. Family data	a. Sexual partner—who does the client have sex with, and have they been tested for HIV; knowledge of procreation in the presence of HIV infection b. Family—health problems of family c. Children—health and HIV status
6. Legal information	a. Health care proxy —who can make decisions (make a copy of the document for records) b. Will—is there one in existence c. Guardianship—who will care for children in case of emergency or death (this may also include any adults for whom the client is responsible)
7. Social data	a. Living arrangements—type and safety of home; egress (elevator, stairs), monthly payments b. Community assessment—safety, grocery stores, pharmacies, delivery available c. Spiritual needs—the importance of religion and spirituality
8. Financial concerns	a. Current employment and any health hazards associated with job (e.g., an HIV-infected nurse who works in a tuberculosis clinic); is there a disability plan b. Income—monthly and annual amount c. Health care payment—insurance and type (indemnity or HMO) d. Eligibility for entitlement—Medicare, Medicaid
9. Agencies providing service	Services from all health or social service agencies

Health Teaching for the Client with HIV Disease

Topic	Encourage	Discourage	Rationale
Stress	A proactive response style to HIV disease Identifying stressor categories (Pivar & Temoshok, 1990): 1. HIV diagnostic testing 2. Severe symptom or illness episodes 3. Treatment issues 4. Complications with family, work, school (or finances) 5. Physical and psychologic limitations or losses 6. Concerns about future Psychoeducational support groups to reduce stress and improve coping (Moulton et al., 1990; Perry et al., 1991) Individual strategies to reduce stress such as: 1. Exercise 2. Meditation 3. Use of visualization 4. Relaxation techniques 5. Use of therapeutic touch	Passive attitude and/or self-destructive behaviors	Stress may negatively affect the immune response and favor progression of HIV-related disease (Evans et al., 1991; Flescher et al., 1992; Hassan & Douglas, 1990).
	Seeking factual information related to HIV disease from knowledgeable health care professionals	Relying on friends, gossip in the media for the "latest" information	
Exercise	A daily schedule of exercise activities	Continuing or adapting a sedentary lifestyle	Exercise may be physiologically, immunologically, and psychologically beneficial to HIV-infected persons and may favorably influence the course of HIV disease (LaPerriene et al., 1990; 1991; MacArthur et al., 1992; Rigsby et al., 1992; Schlenzig et al., 1992).

Topic	Encourage	Discourage	Rationale
Sexual Practices	Safer sexual practices (see Chapter 2)	Unsafe sex	Latex condom use reduces the risk of gonorrhea, herpes simplex virus, genital ulcers, and pelvic inflammatory disease and provides a barrier to HIV, hepatitis B virus, and *Chlamydia trachomatis* (Centers for Disease Control and Prevention [CDC], 1993).
	Proper use of male condoms, including:	Improper use of a male condom, including:	
	1. Using a latex condom only	1. Using natural-membrane condoms	
	2. Using a new condom with each sexual act and/or partner	2. Reusing condom or using same condom for insertive sex when having sex with multiple partners at the same time	
	3. Carefully handling the condom	3. Damaging condom with fingernail, teeth, or other sharp objects	
	4. Putting on the condom before genital contact with partner and when penis is erect	4. Using condom only for vaginal or anal penetration or attempting to apply condom to a flaccid penis	
	5. Ensuring that no air is trapped in tip of condom	5. Leaving air bubble at tip of condom	
	6. Ensuring adequate lubrication during vaginal or anal intercourse	6. Engaging in "dry" intercourse	
	7. Using only water-based lubricants (e.g., K-Y jelly, glycerine) with latex condom	7. Using oil-based lubricants (e.g., petroleum jelly, shortening, mineral oil, massage oils, body lotions, or cooking oil), which can weaken latex	
	8. Holding the condom firmly against base of penis during withdrawal and withdrawing penis while still erect	8. Allowing slippage or spillage when withdrawing	
	9. Storing of condoms in a cool, dry place, away from direct sunlight	9. Using damaged condoms, as evidenced by brittleness, stickiness, or discoloration	
	10. Checking expiration date	10. Using outdated condoms	

Topic	Encourage	Discourage	Rationale
Sexual Practices—*con't*	Proper use of the female condom; second choice to male latex condom	Improper use of the female condom	The female condom has limited information available on its effectiveness in preventing sexually transmitted diseases, and has a relatively high pregnancy rate (26%) (Food and Drug Administration, 1993).
	Use of nonoxynol-9 (a nonionic surfactant spermicide); no studies have shown that the use of nonoxynol-9, used with a condom, increases the protection provided by use of a latex condom alone (CDC, 1993)		
	Use of barrier protection for fellatio and cunnilingus (condoms and dental dams)	Performing fellatio or cunnilingus without a barrier	
	Using latex gloves for digital insertive manipulative practices	Inserting finger(s) into vagina or rectum without a barrier	
Procreation	Providing unbiased information regarding HIV disease so that client can make informed reproductive decisions, including (Berman, 1993; Smeltzer & Whipple, 1991):	Negating the fact that the client does have reproductive options	Through counseling the client may achieve sufficient knowledge to make informed choices about procreation (Berman, 1993).
	1. Illness may occur in the mother during pregnancy, and choices regarding treatment will have to be made that may be toxic to the fetus 2. The HIV status of the child may not be known until 15 months after birth 3. Either the child or the mother, or both, may become ill and die		Maternal antibodies are found in a child's blood for 12 to 15 months after birth. A new test to identify infected newborn infants accurately by 3 months of age is available, but not yet in widespread use (Miles et al., 1993).

Topic	Encourage	Discourage	Rationale
Procreation—*con't*	Additional considerations— 1. Possible illness and death of the father 2. Finances 3. Support systems 4. Guardianship and adoption Choices including 1. Contraception 2. Abortion		
Nutrition	Increased intake of protein (fish, chicken, meat, eggs, milk, cheese, dried beans, nuts, and tofu) Increased intake of carbohydrates as a source of calories (bread, cereals, rice, macaroni, noodles, potatoes, dried beans, plantain, fruits, cakes, cookies, and candy) Increased intake of fat (butter, margarine, oils, mayonnaise, salad dressing, cheese, sour cream, whole milk, sausages, salami, bacon, bologna, and other cold, high-fat meats, and cold cuts)	Diets that are inadequate in protein intake Diets that are calorically sparse	Nutritional counseling and support can improve the nutritional status of people (Beach, 1992; Bradley-Springer, 1991; Kotler, 1992). High nutrient intake is associated with higher $CD4^{+}$ T-cell counts and can reduce the rate of AIDS development (Abrams et al., 1993).
	Increased vitamin and mineral intake by taking a multivitamin daily and eating the above-mentioned foods as well as fruits and vegetables Increased intake of water and juices on a daily basis Participation in meal programs for people with HIV disease as an opportunity to learn more about nutrition as well as socialize	Inadequate intake of vitamins and minerals	
	Building on the client's current dietary patterns	Introduction of an entirely new menu or standardized menus that may be irrelevant to the client	

Topic	Encourage	Discourage	Rationale
Food Safety	Prevention of food-borne diseases (CDC, 1989a; Life Sciences Research Office, 1990) by: 1. Eating and drinking pasteurized dairy products (only) 2. Cooking meats, fish, and poultry to "well done" 3. Considering all animal-derived foods as contaminated, and: a. Washing hands immediately after handling b. Using meat thermometer to ensure thorough cooking c. Cooking to achieve internal temperatures of 165° F for poultry and stuffed meats; 150° F for pork, and at least 140° F for other foods (Nadakavukaren, 1990) d. Using separate cutting boards for raw and cooked foods 4. For microwave cooking, following directions carefully, especially standing time, which allows heat to fully penetrate food 5. When barbecuing, precooking meat first (especially chicken) 6. Washing utensils used for meats before reuse or before use on other foods 7. Wearing disposable gloves if there are cuts or abrasions on hands 8. Washing all fruits and vegetables thoroughly before eating 9. When food shopping:	The nine factors most often implicated in bacterial food poisoning (Nadakavukaren, 1990, p. 219) 1. Eating of raw protein foods, such as uncooked eggs, rare meat, and sushi 2. Failure to refrigerate foods properly 3. Preparing food a day or more before it is to be served 4. Failure to cook foods thoroughly 5. Poor personal hygiene when handling food 6. Improper "hot" holding (keeping foods in heating trays at temperatures under 140° F) 7. Inadequate reheating of cooked foods 8. Failure to avoid moldy or spoiled foods 9. Use of foods after labeled expiration date	Infectious complications can be prevented by avoiding ingestion of contaminated food (Filice & Pomeroy, 1991).

Topic	Encourage	Discourage	Rationale
Food Safety—*con't*	a. Placing raw meat or poultry into plastic bags to prevent juices from leaking onto other foods b. Reading expiration or "sell by" dates and pasteurized labels c. Refrigerating perishables as soon as possible		
Water Safety	At home, use of boiled water for drinking or boiling of unsafe water for 10 minutes to sterilize it (CDC, 1990)		Infectious complications can be prevented by avoiding ingestion of contaminated water (Filice & Pomeroy, 1991).
	When away from home, drinking bottled or canned carbonated water or soft drinks	Adding ice cubes to drinks	Water-borne diseases continue to occur from relatively sophisticated community water systems (CDC, 1991; Gold, 1993).
	After using swimming pools, hot tubs or whirlpools, showering well and using an antimicrobial soap	Swallowing water during recreational activities	Water-borne diseases can occur as a result of surface contact with or swallowing contaminated water (CDC, 1991).
Skin Care	Keeping skin moist and intact (Hardy, 1992) Showering daily for at least 10 minutes Maintaining water temperature of 90° to 105° F Using a superfatted soap Patting skin dry and, while damp, applying an emollient cream	Tub baths Using drying, perfumed soap Using creams and lotions that have a high alcohol content and are drying	Secondary skin infections or transfer of infections from one part of the body to another can be prevented and the effects of xerosis (dry skin) and ichthyosis (rough, thick, scaly skin), the most common dermatoses seen in HIV infection minimized (Duvic, 1991).
Hair Care	Washing hair infrequently Using mild soap Using conditioner Covering head while in bed Combing hair	Washing hair daily Using drying, perfumed shampoo Brushing hair	Hair loss related to telogen effluvium (decrease in number of hair follicles), caused by severe stress, recurrent infections, and high fevers can be minimized (Cockerell, 1991).

Topic	Encourage	Discourage	Rationale
Mouth Care	Using a soft toothbrush	Using firm or hard toothbrush	The incidence and/or severity of secondary oral infections, especially thrush, can be reduced.
	Using nonabrasive toothpaste (or baking soda)	Using abrasive toothpaste	
	Brushing surface of teeth only		
	Using Toothettes for mucosal surface cleaning	Brushing mucosal surfaces	
	Performing mouth care t.i.d.	Performing mouth care only q.d. or b.i.d.	
Hand Washing	Washing frequently after activities of daily living	Using hot water	Secondary infections related to poor hand-washing practices can be prevented.
	Using soap in a pump dispenser	Using bar soap	
	Rinsing well		
	Applying emollient cream to protect the skin		
	Wearing rubber or latex gloves when cleaning		
	Demonstrating hand washing	Teaching hand washing without demonstrating correct method	
Environmental Cleaning and Safety	Using household bleach (5.25% sodium hypochlorite) diluted; $\frac{1}{4}$ cup of bleach per gallon of tap water (CDC, 1989b)	Using expensive ineffective (for disinfection) household detergents	Secondary infections related to unclean environment and contamination of environment with HIV can be prevented.
	Discarding solution daily and remixing when necessary	Using cleaning solutions beyond 24 hours after mixing	
	Cleaning up blood or body fluids with this solution		
	Using household bleach for laundry soiled with blood or body fluids		
	Using securely fastened plastic bags to discard disposable items contaminated with blood or body fluids	Discarding soiled disposable items without using secured bags	
	Placing used needles and sharps in puncture-resistant containers such as detergent containers or coffee cans (United States Environmental Protection Agency, 1990)	Throwing used needles and sharps directly into household garbage	

Topic	Encourage	Discourage	Rationale
Environmental Cleaning and Safety—*con't*	Cleaning or changing air conditioner filters frequently		
Pet Care	Having pet care performed by someone other than person with HIV disease When necessary, wearing gloves and washing hands when finished Always washing hands, face, etc., after having direct contact with body secretions or excretions from pets or when scratched Keeping domestic pets, especially cats, indoors	Handling pet excreta or cleaning litter boxes, bird cages, or aquariums	Certain infectious complications that are zoonotic can be prevented (Filice & Pomeroy, 1991).
	Feeding only commercially prepared canned or dry pet food and meats that are cooked thoroughly	Feeding raw meat or poultry to domestic animals	
Alcohol Drinking	Abstinence or modification	Regular consumption of alcohol	Although Kaslow and colleagues (1989) found no effect on the progression of HIV disease, Bagasara and associates (1993) found that alcohol intake did increase HIV replication.
Smoking	Reduction in smoking Avoidance of smoking Or starting a smoking cessation program	Continued smoking Returning to smoking as a means of coping with stress	Smoking may negatively influence the course of HIV disease and increase the propensity for development of pulmonary opportunistic infections, oral mucosal lesions, and periodontal disease (Buskin et al., 1992; Clarke et al., 1993; Forthal et al., 1992; Neiman et al., 1993; Royce & Winkelstein, 1990; Swango et al., 1991).

Topic	Encourage	Discourage	Rationale
Intravenous Drug Use	Cessation of drug use and referral for treatment Not sharing drug paraphernalia with others Disinfecting drug paraphernalia before sharing equipment (if client persists in sharing) Open dialogue regarding continued drug use Referral to needle exchange program (if locally available)	Sharing of contaminated drug paraphernalia Client and health care professional avoiding discussion of drug use	Prevent transmission of blood-borne disease. Cessation of intravenous drug use may result in slowing of HIV disease progression (Weber et al., 1990).
Travel	Travel planning	Travel to middle, central, and south central United States, including the Ohio and Mississippi river basins, as well as the Caribbean and South America (to avoid histoplasmosis); travel to Arizona, California, Nevada, New Mexico, Utah, and western Texas, as well as Mexico and Central and South America (to avoid coccidiomycosis)	Prevent opportunistic infections (Jewett & Hecht, 1993).
	Nutrition safety 1. Cooking all meat, fish, poultry, and eggs well done and served hot 2. Eating only fresh fruits and vegetables that can be peeled 3. Drinking only bottled water or canned carbonated water or soft drinks 4. Purchasing food in restaurants or hotels	1. Eating undercooked or raw meat, fish, poultry, or eggs 2. Eating prepared fruits and vegetables that are not cooked (e.g. salads) 3. Adding ice cubes to drinks (even to alcoholic drinks) 4. Buying food from street vendors	
	Planning for special needs 1. Requesting in advance a room with a refrigerator (for medication storage), a request honored by most hotels	1. Waiting until checking in to request the special need	

Topic	Encourage	Discourage	Rationale
Travel—*con't*	2. Requesting a wheelchair in advance for movement into and out of airports, as well as for transfers between connecting flights	2. Waiting until arriving at an airport to request wheelchair transport	
	Consulting with a health care provider before traveling to discuss the possible need for chemoprophylaxis for traveler's diarrhea		Prevent gastrointestinal infection (DuPont & Erickson, 1993).
Health Care Follow-Up	Establishing a pattern for health care follow-up (e.g., physician, nurse practitioner, visiting nurse, clinic)	Changing patterns of health care follow-up	Patients with CD4+ T-cell counts greater than 500 cells/mm^3 can be reassured that they are at the same risk for developing any pathologic condition as HIV-negative person and can handle most minor symptomatic problems without professional consultation. Patients with declining CD4+ counts less than 500 cells/mm^3, should be taught signs and symptoms that may indicate serious disease (Hecht & Soloway, 1993).
	Establishing a relationship with health care professional knowledgeable about HIV disease	Seeking health care from professionals with knowledge deficits of HIV disease	
	Watching for signs and symptoms indicating secondary complications of HIV disease including but not limited to: 1. Skin lesions, rashes, itching, lumps or bruising 2. Lesions or exudate in mouth 3. Persistent fever, night sweats 4. Extreme fatigue even when getting plenty of rest 5. Weight loss 6. Changes in digestion, difficulty in swallowing, and diarrhea 7. Shortness of breath, persistent coughing 8. Headache, visual changes, numbness in arms and legs, forgetfulness, dizziness, seizures 9. Unusual bleeding (e.g., bleeding gums)	Ignoring warning signs	

Topic	Encourage	Discourage	Rationale
Additional Considerations	Receiving TB testing and influenza vaccination annually		
	Using own personal care items (e.g., razors, toothbrushes, makeup)	Sharing personal care items	
	Refraining from donating blood or organs	Donating blood or making plans to donate body organs	
	Informing health care professionals responsible for primary care that the client has HIV disease	Withholding information about HIV disease from health care professionals responsible for coordinating care	Preventing transmissions and withholding information on current HIV diagnosis could result in a delay in diagnosing and treating problems related to HIV disease.
	Planning financially	Waiting until a crisis occurs to access entitlements	

References

Abrams, B., Duncan. D., Hertz-Picaotto, I. (1993). A prospective study of dietary intake and acquired immune deficiency syndrome in HIV seropositive homosexual men. *Journal of Acquired Immune Deficiency Syndrome, 6*(8), 949-958.

Bagasra, O., Kajdacsy-Balla, A., Lischner, H.W., et al. (1993). Alcohol intake increases human immunodeficiency virus type I replication in human peripheral blood mononuclear cells. *Journal of Infectious Diseases, 167*(4), 789-797.

Beach, R.S. (1992). Nutrition and people with HIV/AIDS: A summary for data presented at the VIII International Conference on AIDS. *Nutrition and HIV/AIDS, 1*(1), 107-108.

Berman, N. (1993). Family and reproductive issues: Reproductive counseling. *AIDS Clinical Care, 5*(6), 45-47.

Bradley-Springer, L. (1991). Nutrition and support in HIV infection: A multilevel analysis. *Image: Journal of Nursing Scholarship, 23*(3), 155-159.

Buskin, S.E., Hopkins, S.G., Farizo, K.M. (1992). Heavy smoking increases the risk of *Pneumocystis carinii* pneumonia (PCP). *International Conference on AIDS* (abstract No. WeC1030), *8*(1), We50.

Centers for Disease Control (1989a). *Eating defensively: Food safety advice for persons with AIDS.* (videorecording). Atlanta: CDC.

Centers for Disease Control (1989b). Guidelines for prevention of transmission of human immunodeficiency virus and hepatitis B virus to health care and public safety workers. *Morbidity and Mortality Weekly Report, 38*(S-6), 1-37.

Centers for Disease Control (1990). *Health information for international travel.* (HHS Pub. No. CDC 90-8280). Washington, DC: U.S. Government Printing Office.

Centers for Disease Control (1991). Waterborne-disease outbreaks. *Morbidity and Mortality Weekly Report, 40*(SS-3), 1-13.

Centers for Disease Control and Prevention (1993). Update: Barrier protection against HIV infection and other sexually transmitted diseases. *Morbidity and Mortality Weekly Report, 42*(30), 589-591, 597.

Clarke, J.R., Taylor. I.K., Fleming, J. (1993). The epidemiology of HIV-1 infection in the lung in AIDS patients. *AIDS, 7*(4), 555-560.

Cockerell, C.J. (1991). Noninfectious inflammatory skin diseases in HIV-infected individuals. *Dermatologic Clinics, 9*(3), 531-541.

DuPont, H.L., Ericsson, C.D. (1993). Prevention and treatment of traveler's diarrhea. *The New England Journal of Medicine, 328*(25), 1821-1827.

Duvic, M. (1991). Papulosquamous disorders associated with human immunodeficiency virus infection. *Dermatologic Clinics, 9*(3), 523-530.

Evans, D.L., Lesserman, J., Perkins, D.O., et al. (1991). Stress related reduction of natural killer cells in HIV. *International Conference on AIDS.* (abstract No. TH.B. 91), *7*(2), 79.

Filice, G.A., Pomeroy, C. (1991). Preventing secondary infections among HIV-positive persons. *Public Health Report, 106*(5), 503-517.

Flescher, M., Watkins, L.R., Lockwood, L.L., et al. (1992). Specific changes in lymphocyte subpopulations: A potential mechanism for stress-induced immunomodulation. *Journal of Neuroimmunology, 41*(2), 131-142.

Food and Drug Administration (1993). Female condom approval. *FDA Medical Bulletin, 23*(2), 4.

Forthal, D., Gordon, R., Larsen, R. (1992). Cigarette smoking increases the risk of developing cryptococcal meningitis. *International Conference on AIDS.* (abstract No. PoB 3172), *8*(2), B115.

Gold, D. (1993). Treatment briefs: Risky drinking water. *Treatment Issues: The Gay Men's Health Crisis Newsletter of Experimental AIDS Therapies, 7*(7), 6.

Hardy, M.A. (1992). Dry skin care. In G.M. Bulechek & J.A. McCloskey (Eds.), *Nursing interventions: Essential nursing treatments* (2nd ed.) (pp. 34-47). Philadelphia: W.B. Saunders.

Hassan, N.F., Douglas, S.D. (1990). Stress-related neuroimmunomodulation of monocyte-macrophage functions in HIV-1 infection. *Clinical Immunology and Immunopathology, 54*(2), 220-227.

Hecht, F.M., Soloway, B. (1993). Identifying patients at risk for HIV infection. In D.J. Cotton & G.H. Friedland (Eds.), *HIV infection: A primary care approach* (rev. ed.) (p. 307). Waltham, MA: Massachusetts Medical Society.

Jewett, J.F., Hecht, F.M. (1993). Preventive health care for adults with HIV infection. *Journal of the American Medical Association, 269*(9), 1144-1153.

Kaslow, R.A., Blackwelder, W.C., Ostrow, D.G., et al. (1989). No evidence for a role of alcohol or other psychoactive drugs accelerating immunodeficiency in HIV-1 positive individuals. A report from the Multicenter AIDS Cohort Study. *Journal of the American Medical Association, 261*(23), 3424-3429.

Kotler, D. P. (1992). Nutritional effects and support in the patient with acquired immunodeficiency syndrome. *Journal of Nutrition, 122*(Suppl. 3), 723-727.

LaPerriere, A.R., Antoni, M. H., Schniederman, N., et al. (1990). Exercise intervention attenuates emotional distress and natural killer cell decrements following notification of positive serologic status for HIV-1. *Biofeedback and Self Regulation, 15*(3), 229-242.

LaPerriere, A.R., Fletcher, M.A., Antoni, M.I., et al. (1991). Aerobic exercise training in an AIDS risk group. *International Journal of Sports Medicine, 12*(Suppl. 1), 552-557.

Life Sciences Research Office, Federation of American Societies for Experimental Biology (1990, November). *Nutrition and HIV infection* (FDA No. 223-88-2124). Washington, DC: Center for Food Safety and Applied Nutrition, Food and Drug Administration, Department of Health and Human Services.

MacArthur, R.D., Levine, S.D., Birk, T.J., et al. (1992). Cardiopulmonary, immunologic and psychologic responses to exercise training in individuals seropositive for HIV. *International Conference on AIDS.* (abstract No. PuB 7327), *8*(3), 103.

Miles, S.A., Balden, E., Megpantay, L., et al., (1993). Rapid serologic testing with immune-complex–dissociated HIV p24 antigen for early detection of HIV infection in neonates. *New England Journal of Medicine, 328*(5), 297-302.

Moulton J.M., Gurbuz, G., Sweet, D., et al. (1990). Outcome evaluation of eight-week educational support groups: Validating the model using control group comparisons. *International Conference on AIDS.* (abstract No. S.B. 400), *6*(3), 186.

Nadakavukaren, A. (1990). *Man and environment: A health perspective* (3rd ed.). Prospect Heights, IL: Waveland Press.

Nieman, R., Fleming, J., Coker, R.J., et al. (1993). The effect of cigarette on the development of AIDS in HIV-1 seropositive individuals. *AIDS, 7*(5), 705-710.

Perry, S., Fishman, B., Jacobsberg, L., et al. (1991). Effectiveness of psychoeducational interventions in reducing emotional distress after human immunodeficiency virus antibody testing. *Archives of General Psychiatry, 48*(2), 143-147.

Pivar, I., Temoshok, L. (1990). Coping strategies and response styles in homosexual symptomatic seropositive men. *International Conference on AIDS.* (abstract No. S.B. 382), *6*(3), 181.

Rigsby, L.W., Dishman, R.K., Jackson, A.W., et al. (1992). Effects of exercise training on men seropositive for the human immunodeficiency virus- 1. *Medicine and Science in Sports and Exercise, 24*(1), 6-12.

Royce, R.A., Winkelstein, W. (1990). HIV infection, cigarette smoking and CD4+ T-lymphocyte counts: Preliminary results from the San Francisco men's health study. *AIDS, 4*(4), 327-333.

Schlenzig, C., Jaeger, H., Wehrenberg, M., et al. (1992). Physical exercise favorably influences the course of illness in patients with HIV and AIDS. *International Conference on AIDS.* (abstract No. PoB 3401), *8*(2), B153.

Smeltzer, S.C., Whipple, B. (1991). Women and HIV infection. *Image: Journal of Nursing Scholarship, 23*(4), 249-256.

Swango, P.A., Kleinman, P.V., Konzelman, J.L. (1991). HIV and periodontal health. A study of military personnel with HIV. *Journal of the American Dental Association, 122*(8), 49-54.

United States Environmental Protection Agency (1990, January). *Disposal Types for Home Health Care.* (EPA/530-SW-90-014A). Washington, DC: United States Environmental Protection Agency.

Weber, R., Ledergerber, B., Opravil, M., et al. (1990). Progression of HIV infection in misusers of injected drugs who stop injecting or follow a program of maintenance treatment with methadone. *British Medical Journal, 301*(6765), 1362-1365.

(From Flaskerud, J.H. & Ungvarski, P. J. [1995]. HIV/AIDS: A guide to nursing care [3rd ed.]. *Philadelphia: W. B. Saunders.)*

Important Aspects of Antiretroviral Medication Teaching

Background

Experience with drugs used to treat HIV infection has raised concern over the issue of subtherapeutic levels of drugs (insufficient amount of the drug in the blood to maintain its effectiveness) and the development of drug resistance (the drug no longer works effectively against HIV). In many instances this can be avoided if the patient is taught how to take the medications properly.

Points to Emphasize

1. If the directions are to take the medicine with food, take it immediately after eating a full meal.
2. If the directions are to take it on an empty stomach, take it one hour before or two hours after eating a meal.
3. Follow storage instructions and either keep at room temperature or in the refrigerator as directed.
4. It is best, and in some instances necessary, to keep the medicine in the original container.
5. Never adjust (decrease or increase) the prescribed dose. If, for any reason, the client does not wish to take the medicine, he/she should inform the physician or nurse practitioner before doing so.
6. Report any and all side effects of the medicine to the physician or nurse practitioner.
7. Many of these medicines interact with other medicines. Always check with the physician, nurse practitioner, or pharmacist before taking any other medicines (this includes over-the-counter medicines).
8. The client should not change the hours he/she takes the medicines. It is important to space these drugs at specified intervals in order to maintain good blood levels of the drug.
9. Do not share, sell, or give away the medicine.
10. This medicine will not prevent the client from spreading HIV through sex, needle sharing, or through blood/body fluids, so he/she must continue to practice safer sex, avoid sharing needles, exchanging body fluids, etc., in order to prevent HIV transmission.

CHAPTER

28

Nursing Care of Clients with Connective Tissue Disorders

Objectives

28.1 Discuss autoimmunity as it relates to autoimmune disease.
28.2 Discuss the hypotheses related to the etiology of rheumatoid arthritis.
28.3 Describe the pathologic changes in the joint that occur with rheumatoid arthritis.
28.4 Describe physical and laboratory findings (diagnostic criteria) with rheumatoid arthritis.
28.5 Identify the main intervention goals for clients with arthritis.
28.6 Discuss management for clients with arthritis.
28.7 Administer medications prescribed to decrease inflammation and reduce pain with knowledge of the action, toxicity, and nursing considerations of each medication.
28.8 Discuss types and characteristics of unproven remedies for arthritis.
28.9 Describe types of surgical procedures used in the treatment of arthritis.
28.10 Discuss the etiology and pathophysiology of systemic lupus erythematosus.
28.11 Describe physical assessment findings with systemic lupus erythematosus.
28.12 Describe laboratory findings with systemic lupus erythematosus.
28.13 Discuss interventions for clients with systemic lupus erythematosus.

Facilitating Student Learning

CLASSROOM

Class Assignments

- Divide the class into thirds to do literature reviews from the latest publications on one of the following three topics: 1) current research in the area of autoimmune disorders, 2) development of improved methods of total joint replacement, 3) the association of breast implants with connective tissue disorders. Ask students to be prepared to share their findings in class or clinical conference.
- Assign students to use their pharmacology text and prepare drug cards on medications commonly used in the treatment of rheumatoid arthritis.
- Encourage students to visit the Arthritis Foundation to learn the goals and work of the Foundation, and to see materials available for teaching and helping people with arthritis.
- Assign students to complete the activities in the Study Guide for this chapter.

Lecture/Discussion

- Compare and contrast rheumatoid and osteoarthritis. Transparencies 24(T) and 25(T) may be used.
- Discuss nursing diagnoses and appropriate interventions for clients with arthritis. Transparency 26(T) may be used when teaching exercises for clients with arthritis. Since students will have studied the pharmacologic treatment of arthritis when they prepared their drug cards, invite them to participate in the discussion of medication prescribed to decrease inflammation and reduce pain.
- Discuss connective tissue disorders and use systemic lupus erythematosus as an example.

Transparencies

- 24(T)—Rheumatoid Arthritis
- 25(T)—Osteoarthritis
- 26(T)—Exercises for Arthritic People

Guest Speakers

- Invite an orthopedic surgeon to discuss the latest developments in surgical treatment of arthritis.
- Invite physical and occupational therapists to discuss various therapies currently used for clients with arthritis.
- Invite a representative of the Arthritis Foundation to discuss the Foundation's goals and accomplishments.

CLINICAL

Skills Laboratory

- Assign pairs of students to teach each other exercises helpful for arthritic clients to increase flexibility, improve circulation and muscle tone, and prevent further movement restriction.

Clinical Site Activities

- Assign students in the acute care setting to provide care for clients with the various connective tissue disorders discussed in class. Expect the students to individualize the standardized care plans and to consider the person's home environment.
- Arrange for students to accompany the clients to whom they are assigned to the operating and recovery rooms so the students may observe surgical treatment of arthritis.
- In cooperation with community health faculty, arrange for students to provide follow-up care for clients with arthritis after they are discharged from the acute care facility.

Clinical Conference Activities

- Invite several people with arthritis to discuss how they have adapted to the changes in their lifestyles necessitated by arthritis.
- Discuss how alterations in body image (for example, with arthritis or scleroderma) can affect clients with connective tissue disorders, and nursing interventions that may be helpful.
- Ask students to share findings from their literature reviews.
- Ask students to share how they needed to individualize standardized care plans.

Critical Points to Emphasize

- These disorders often occur during young adulthood, impairing mobility and functional capacity.
- Many of the connective tissue disorders are difficult to diagnose as they are characterized by remissions and exacerbations, and have many overlapping signs and symptoms because connective tissue throughout the body may be affected.
- Nursing interventions are aimed primarily at pain control and maintenance of joint mobility.
- Being understanding of the psychosocial effect yet teaching the client to manage self-care is of prime importance.

CHAPTER

29

Structure and Function of the Nervous System

OBJECTIVES

29.1 Describe a neuron, its basic parts, and how it functions.

29.2 Give the general functions of each of the three divisions of the nervous system: central, peripheral, and autonomic.

29.3 List the main parts of the brain with their major functions.

29.4 Name the coverings of the brain and spinal cord, and describe their functions.

29.5 Describe the functions of the cerebrospinal fluid and the blood-brain barrier.

29.6 Describe the reflex arc and how it functions.

29.7 Describe a plexus, and locate and name the major plexuses of the spinal nerves.

29.8 List the names and functions of the cranial nerves.

29.9 Describe the main parts of the autonomic nervous system and how they function.

Facilitating Student Learning

CLASSROOM

Review Activity

- The objectives listed for this chapter are considered review items for students in the nursing major. These objectives can be shared with students to focus their review.

Lecture/Discussion

- Ask students to recall or review from their anatomy and physiology course the functions of the three main divisions of the nervous system. Transparency 29(T) may be used.
- Help students gain an understanding of the functioning of the autonomic nervous system by using a "flight or fight" situation and discussing the effects on various parts of the body. For example, ask the students to pretend they are in the jungle at night where a hungry tiger is on the prowl. (Pupils dilate so they can see better; bronchioles and coronary arteries dilate and heart rate is increased to increase the amount of oxygen to the brain so the ability to think increases; etc.) Refer students to Table 29–5 "Effects of the Sympathetic and Parasympathetic Nervous Systems" in Chapter 29 of the text.
- Discuss the importance of understanding the origins of the cranial nerves in relation to neuro checks. Refer students to Table 29–4 "Functions and Types of Cranial Nerves" in Chapter 27 of the text and Transparency 31(T) may be used.
- Discuss the importance of understanding the anatomy of the motor and sensory tracts in relation to spinal cord injuries. This is of special importance when there is only a part of the spinal cord injured and not complete transsection of the cord.

Transparencies

- 29(T)—Organization of the Nervous System
- 31(T)—Distribution of Cranial Nerves

CLINICAL

Clinical Site Activity

- With each patient assignment on the neuro unit, ask students to compare normal anatomy and physiology with the pathophysiology.

CHAPTER

30

Assessment of Clients with Neurologic Disorders

Objectives

30.1 Describe the elements of a neurologic health history.

30.2 Identify the purpose and components of a detailed mental status exam.

30.3 Demonstrate the correct test for each cranial nerve.

30.4 List elements to be assessed in the motor examination.

30.5 Give examples of abnormal motor responses.

30.6 List elements to be assessed in the sensory examination.

30.7 Discuss the relationship between the abnormal sensory or motor response and the portion of the nervous system that is damaged.

30.8 Demonstrate the correct tests for major reflexes.

30.9 Differentiate between upper and lower motor neuron damage.

30.10 Interpret the neurologic implications of each section of the neurologic observation chart.

30.11 Give the diagnostic purposes of common neurologic tests.

30.12 Describe common neurologic diagnostic tests in layman's terminology.

30.13 Identify potential complications of common neurologic diagnostic tests.

30.14 Plan and implement appropriate nursing interventions for people before, during, and after assessment and treatment procedures.

Facilitating Student Learning

CLASSROOM

Review Activity

- Ask students to review Barbara Bates' film on neurologic examination, Part 11, "Neurologic: Cranial Nerves and Sensory System" and Part 12, "Neurologic: Motor System and Reflexes" from Barbara Bates, MD, "A Visual Guide to Physical Examination," 1995.

Lecture/Discussion

- Coordinate abnormal neurologic assessment with a review of normal anatomy and physiology of the nervous system; e.g., patterns of sensory loss with various sensory tracts. Transparencies 30(T), 31(T), 32(T), and 33(T) may be used.
- Discuss the importance of using a neurological observation chart or record when assessing people with neurologic problems.
- Stress the necessity of preparing the client for a neurologic diagnostic test, psychosocially as well as physically. Ask the students to give brief descriptions of some common neurologic tests in layman's terminology and to complete the "At a Glance Worksheet" in the Study Guide. Transparencies 34(T) and 35(T) may be used.

Transparencies

- 31(T)—Major Distribution of Spinal Nerves
- 32(T)—Patterns of Sensory Loss with Brain and Spinal Cord Disorders
- 33(T)—Patterns of Sensory Loss with Peripheral Nerve Lesions
- 34(T)—Cerebral Angiography
- 35(T)—Lumbar Puncture

CLINICAL

Skills Laboratory

- Assign pairs of students to practice neurologic examinations on each other.

Clinical Site Activity

- Arrange for students to accompany clients who are having neurologic diagnostic tests. Instruct students to do preliminary reading about the procedure and required client preparation. During the procedure, students should focus not only on the procedural components but on client comfort, safety, and response to the procedure. Postprocedure, students should assist in giving any specific nursing care required.

Clinical Conference Activities

- During a clinical conference, invite a person with a neurologic disorder to come visit. Demonstrate taking a neurologic history and various components of the neurologic physical examination. Ask the students to interpret the findings.
- Ask students to give a brief presentation of their experiences of observing diagnostic tests and to include nursing care before, during, and after the procedure.

CHAPTER

31

Nursing Care of Comatose or Confused Clients

Objectives

31.1 Differentiate between the etiology and clinical manifestations of two major kinds of physiologic disorders that can produce sustained unconsciousness.

31.2 Identify levels of consciousness and discuss advantages of using a tool like the Glasgow Coma Scale to determine the level of consciousness versus charting descriptions like "unconscious," "obtunded," or "in a deep coma."

31.3 Describe variations in breathing patterns that could indicate neurologic dysfunction.

31.4 Describe six areas of assessment in "neuro checks": level of consciousness, breathing pattern, eye movement, pupillary changes, motor response, vital sign changes.

31.5 Relate the importance of the six components of the "neuro checks" to cerebral functioning.

31.6 Discuss immediate assessment and interventions needed for an unconscious client.

31.7 Plan detailed nursing interventions and set priorities in providing nursing care for the unconscious client.

Facilitating Student Learning

CLASSROOM

Class Assignment

- Assign students to complete the activities in the Study Guide for Chapter 31.

Lecture/Discussion

- Using the illustration of normal and abnormal breathing patterns [Transparency 36(T)], ask students to identify the areas of injury in the brain that correspond to the specific breathing pattern resulting from the injury.
- Give students a set of ABGs; for example, pH 7.15, pO_2 40 mmHg, pCO_2 60 mmHg, HCO_3 21 mEq/L, and ask the students to explain the effect of elevated CO_2 and low O_2 levels on brain function.
- Ask each student to write their definition of "unconscious," "obtunded," "stuperous," "in a deep coma," "confused," "nonresponsive," and "lethargic." Discuss the differences and relate the difficulty in using these words to the advantages of using a tool like the Glasgow Coma Scale when assessing patients with neurologic problems.
- Ask students to imagine they are unconscious. Then, ask them to list the nursing care interventions they would like to receive and to set priorities. Compare lists for similarities and differences.

Transparency

- 36(T)—Respiratory Patterns and Pupil Appearances Associated with Lesions of Various Neurologic Structures

Group Activities

- Divide the class in half. Ask one group to develop a care plan for a client with brain injury and hypothermia. Ask the other group to develop a care plan for a client with brain injury and hyperthermia. In class, compare and contrast the two care plans.

CLINICAL

Clinical Site Activity

- In the clinical area, assign students to clients with altered consciousness.

Clinical Conference Activity

- From the students' clinical experiences in caring for unconscious clients, ask the class to develop a list of common nursing diagnoses and interventions.

Critical Points to Emphasize

PHYSIOLOGIC COMA

Etiology

- Structural lesions (tumors, hemorrhage from trauma, or ruptured aneurysm)
- Metabolic disorders beginning in another system and affecting the brain through hypoxia, ischemia, or accumulation of waste products
- Toxins

Pathophysiology

- Impairment/destruction of reticular activating system
- Reduction of cerebral oxygen
- Accumulation of waste products
- Impaired metabolism of neurons

CLINICAL MANIFESTATIONS

Structural lesions

- *Supratentorial* (above the cerebellum) lesions: symptoms vary depending on area of cerebral hemispheres damaged; e.g., area in right parietal lobe results in numbness in corresponding area on left side of body controlled, intact oculovestibular reflexes
- *Infratentorial* (cerebellum and brain stem) lesions: usually produce coma early, oculovestibular abnormalities, abnormal respiratory patterns, pupillary changes

Metabolic Disorders or Toxins

- Usually produce confusion first, bilateral manifestations (e.g., tremor of both hands), generalized seizures, normal pupillary responses unless drug overdose

Nursing Care

- Apply stiff collar (assume cervical spine injury if trauma present), clear airway and maintain lateral position, hyperventilate, maintain systolic blood pressure between 100–160 mmHg, use IV diazepam (Valium) to control seizures, normalize body temperature, maintain hydration without fluid overload (intake = output, stable body weight), maintain nutrition (enteral or parental feeding prn), use oscillating bed to prevent complications of bedrest, assist with diagnosis and treatment of cause of coma (notify physician of change in neurologic status), stimulate patient to improve prognosis, understand that vigorous treatment is not appropriate with poor prognosis

POOR PROGNOSIS

- Early and sustained absence of pupillary, corneal, or oculovestibular responses, coma lasting > one week with metabolic disorders, assess families for approachability to determine possibility of organ donation

CHAPTER

32

Nursing Care of Clients with Cerebrovascular Disorders

Objectives

32.1 Describe pathophysiology of the following neurologic disorders: increased intracranial pressure (ICP), stroke (CVA), transient ischemia attack (TIA), headaches, traumatic brain injury.

32.2 Identify three common causes of increased ICP.

32.3 Describe the neurologic signs of herniation syndromes.

32.4 List the advantages of increased ICP monitoring.

32.5 Discuss in detail the use of the Glasgow Coma Scale.

32.6 Describe immediate assessment and interventions needed for a client with an onset of increased ICP.

32.7 Identify nursing responsibilities in interventions for clients with increased ICP.

32.8 Recognize the signs and symptoms occurring with the acute phase of stroke, migraine headache, and head injury.

32.9 Implement appropriate measures for individuals with the specific conditions listed in Objective 8.

32.10 Discuss the limitations caused by a stroke and the impact on family caregivers of a person who has had a stroke.

Facilitating Student Learning

CLASSROOM

Class Assignment

- Assign students to complete the activities in the Study Guide for Chapter 32.

Lecture/Discussion

- Using the illustration of normal and abnormal breathing patterns [Transparency 29–1(T)], ask students to identify the areas of injury in the brain that correspond to the specific breathing pattern resulting from the injury.
- Refer students to their basic nursing text to review the concept of inflammation. In class discussion, relate this concept to the pathophysiology of increased ICP. Then, ask students to give the rationale for using steroids as medical treatment for increased ICP.
- Assign students to review the expected changes in vital signs of patients experiencing shock in Chapter 22 of the text. In lecture, contrast these changes in vital signs with changes in vital signs which patients may exhibit with increased ICP. Transparency 211(M) and Transparency 38(M) may be used with this activity.
- Using a model of the brain, demonstrate to students the mechanics of the various herniation syndromes. Ask the students, based on their understanding of the functions of the different areas of the brain, to describe potential signs and symptoms of various herniation syndromes. Transparency 37(T) and Figure 32–3 may be used with this activity.
- Discuss aneurysm precautions and the rationale for each.
- Emphasize the importance of preventing increased ICP. Give students examples of nursing interventions that may be appropriate for some clients but that would be contraindicated for the client who has had a neurosurgical procedure; for example, turning and coughing, nasal suctioning.
- Supply students with case studies of clients with increased ICP. Ask the students to identify the specific crisis, give emergency interventions, and rationale for the interventions. The case study in Chapter 32 of the Study Guide can be used as an example.

Transparencies

- 37(T)—Mechanics of Tentorial Herniation
- 38(M)—Physical Changes with Increased Intracranial Pressure
- 39(T)—Events Causing Stroke
- 40(T)—Mechanisms of Head Injury
- 41(T)—Formation of Hematoma After Head Injury

Guest Speaker

- Invite to class a speech pathologist who works with clients who have had strokes. Ask the students to share the communication difficulties they have encountered while working with stroke victims so the speech pathologist may help the students with nursing interventions.

CLINICAL

Clinical Site Activities

- In the clinical area, assign students to clients with increased ICP or the potential for developing ICP.
- Arrange for students to accompany the clients to whom they have been assigned to the operating room to observe endarterectomy and extracranial-intracranial bypass surgeries.
- Arrange clinical experiences with a home healthcare agency so students may participate in home care of clients with neurologic disorders. Ask students to collect data that would reflect promotion of the person's independence in all aspects of care; e.g.., decision-making, modification of home environment.
- Ask students to participate in interdisciplinary discharge planning conferences for clients with neurologic disorders in acute care settings.
- Ask students to collaborate with the primary nurse in completing discharge summary forms on clients with neurologic disorders.

Clinical Conference Activities

- Assign groups of students to visit the American Heart Association to obtain client education materials regarding prevention of stroke and rehabilitation of the client who has had a CVA. Obtain Clinical Practice Guidelines developed by the Agency for Healthcare Policy and Research (AHCPR) on poststroke rehabilitation. Discuss the materials in clinical conference.
- Ask a student to lead a client care conference to identify nursing diagnoses and interventions appropriate for a client having an endarterectomy or an extracranial-intracranial bypass.

Critical Points to Emphasize

INCREASED INTRACRANIAL PRESSURE (ICP)

- *Etiology*: hemorrhage, tumor, hydrocephalus, cerebral infraction, abscess, toxin
- *Pathophysiology*: expansion of brain tissue, increase in blood or cerebrospinal fluid within skull which cannot expand
- *Herniation*: displacement of brain tissue, occurs late in increased ICP, body's last attempt to adapt, always an emergency regardless of type
- *Clinical Manifestations*: subtle changes that vary with each patient, most important change is any alteration in level of consciousness
- *Signs*: include restlessness, irritability, confusion, decrease in Glasgow Coma Scale score, changes in speech or vision, abnormal pupillary reactions, motor or sensory changes, changes in cardiac rate or rhythm, nausea or vomiting, headache, increase in systolic blood pressure with a widening pulse pressure, decreasing respirations, abnormal breathing patterns, changes in body temperature
- *Emergency Care*: airway maintenance, intubation with oxygenation ($pO_2 > 90$ mmHg) and hyperventilation, osmotic diuretics (Mannitol IV), steroids (Decadron IV), elevation of head (30°), sedate prn (Versed IV), drain cerebrospinal fluid (keep ICP < 20), maintain fluid status (normal serum sodium and osmolality)

CVA

- *Etiology*: occlusion (thrombus-atherosclerotic plaque or embolus) or hemorrhage (hypertension or aneurysm causing rupture of vessel) resulting in brain ischemia and infarct
- *Pathophysiology*: decreased blood supply, hypoxia, ischemia, infarction
- *Clinical Manifestations*: transient ischemia attacks (TIAs)—early warning signs of stroke caused by thrombus, headache, dizziness, fainting, paresthesias, and nosebleed may precede hemorrhage in hypertensive clients, no warning signs with emboli, signs must persist longer than 24 hours to be diagnostic of stroke (vary depending on area of brain damaged and include hemiparesis and hemiplegia, apraxia, aphasia, dysphagia, visual changes, agnosia, kinesthesia, abstract thought changes, emotional lability, incontinence)
- *Emergency Care*: airway maintenance, turn patient on side if unconscious, loosen shirt collar, elevate head, avoid neck flexion, keep quiet
- *Critical Care*: hypervolemic hemodilution, anticoagulant if hemorrhage is not cause, fibrinolytic inhibitor aminocaproic acid (Amicar) if hemorrhage is cause, edema and seizure and B/P control
- *Aneurysm Precautions*: dim lights, limit visitation, decrease noise, private room, elevate head of bed, avoid Valsalva maneuver, administer analgesics (codeine) and sedatives (Phenobarbital)
- *Acute and Subacute Care*: multidisciplinary services such as physical, occupational, and speech therapy
- *Nursing Care*:

  —assess prn and report changes indicative of increased ICP

  —maintain airway and prevent aspiration

  —increase mobility (exercises, wheelchair, braces, physical therapy)

  —maintain normal body temperature

  —protect skin

  —prevent corneal abrasion (eye patch and artificial tears prn)

—prevent contractures, "frozen shoulder," foot drop (range of motion exercises, position with joints in extension, arm sling prn, hightop tennis shoes)

—be patient and encourage self-care (teach family the importance)

—prevent injury from falls and burns

—provide adequate nutrition (use feeding principles for clients with dysphagia)

—use communication techniques for clients with aphasia

—provide orientation

—be understanding and kind

- *Community and Self-Care*: use individualized unit-dose containers and medication charts to help clients learn self-medication, provide list of specific community resources, use rehabilitation home visits to assess client's ability to be mobile at home and use home appliances

BRAIN INJURIES

- *Etiology*: sudden force to head (blunt or penetrating trauma)
- *Pathophysiology*: concussion (no visible damage, biochemical damage), contusion (bruise), hematoma (bleeding) that may be epidural or subdural
- *Clinical Manifestations*: concussion results in loss of consciousness for five minutes or less, contusions and hematomas cause brain damage, signs of cerebral contusion vary depending on area of brain affected, brain stem injuries usually render a client immediately unresponsive with respiratory, pupillary, eye movement, and motor abnormalities. Clients may have CSF leak from nose or ear, blood behind tympanic membrane, periorbital ecchymoses, bruise over mastoid (Battle's sign) with basilar skull fracture. Epidural hematoma usually produces unconsciousness shortly after injury, brief period of recovery, and then rapid deterioration into coma. Subdural hematomas may be acute or chronic with the acute type producing symptoms similar to epidural hematomas.
- *Emergency Care*: assume cervical spine injury and treat accordingly until lateral cervical spine radiographs are obtained, cover head wounds, do not attempt to remove penetrating objects, ventilatory support
- *Critical Care*: continue ventilatory support, observe for increasing ICP and control (see ICP above), observe for and treat diabetes insipidus or syndrome of inappropriate secretion of antidiuretic hormone (SIADH), neurogenic pulmonary edema which is similar to adult respiratory distress syndrome (ARDS)
- *Recovery Phase*: Observe for posttraumatic response and be supportive

CHAPTER

33

Nursing Care of Clients with Cerebral Disorders

Objectives

33.1 Identify pathophysiology of the following neurologic disorders: seizures, tumors, and infections.

33.2 Relate the signs and symptoms of the above listed disorders to the pathophysiology by recalling normal functioning of the neuroanatomy involved.

33.3 Discuss the nursing interventions for the nursing diagnosis Potential for injury due to generalized seizure.

33.4 Discuss the social stigma that continues to be attached to a diagnosis of epilepsy.

33.5 Discuss the action, side effects, and nursing implications for medications given to treat epilepsy.

33.6 Discuss interdisciplinary management of the patient with an intracranial tumor.

33.7 List items to be included in the preoperative preparation for intracranial surgery that are different from those for general surgery.

33.8 Identify the potential intraoperative complications with intracranial surgery.

33.9 Utilize nursing care plans in caring for clients who have had intracranial surgery to prevent complications postoperatively.

33.10 Give rationale for nursing interventions for clients having intracranial surgery.

Facilitating Student Learning

CLASSROOM

Class Assignment

- Ask students to prepare from their text a summary of the neurologic disorders, including definition, pathophysiology, usual signs and symptoms, diagnostic tests, and usual nursing care. Use this written assignment as a basis for class discussion.

Lecture/Discussion

- Stress the importance of maintaining a patent airway during status epilepticus. Ask students to identify how they would assess the respiratory status during status epilepticus, and give nursing interventions for maintaining a patent airway.
- Emphasize the changes in societal attitudes and in law that affect persons with epilepsy. Include nursing strategies that will help the client accept a diagnosis of epilepsy.
- Discuss aneurysm precautions and the rationale for each.
- Explain structures involved in neurosurgical procedures. Transparency 42(T) may be used to explain pituitary surgeries.
- Give standard positioning for clients postintracranial surgery and stress why these positions should not be changed without a physician's order.
- Emphasize the importance of preventing increased intracranial pressure. Give students examples of nursing interventions that may be appropriate for some clients but which would be contraindicated for the client who has had a neurosurgical procedure; for example, turning and coughing, nasal suctioning.
- Discuss the extra-meticulous handwashing and aseptic technique necessary when doing dressing changes or emptying suction drains on clients who have had intracranial surgery.
- Discuss the importance of maintaining continuous suction by keeping suction reservoirs emptied on clients who have had intracranial surgery. Use Transparency 43(T).

Transparencies

- 42(T)—Neurosurgical Procedures: Pituitary Surgery
- 43(T)—Neurosurgical Suction Drain

CLINICAL

Clinical Site Activities

- Ask students to use the textbook summary of the neurologic disorder and compare the "textbook picture" with the clients to whom they have been assigned.
- Ask students to adapt the standardized plans they have located or developed to the clients to whom they have been assigned.
- Ask students to give the rationales for specific nursing interventions they have included in the nursing care plan for clients with neurologic disorders.
- Arrange for students to accompany clients who are having neurosurgery to the operating and recovery rooms.
- If possible, arrange for each student to provide pre- and postoperative care for a client having a neurosurgical procedure.

Clinical Conference Activity

- Assign groups of students to visit the American Heart Association and the Epilepsy Foundation to obtain client education materials. Have students share the materials in clinical conference.

CHAPTER

34

Nursing Care of Clients with Degenerative Neurologic Disorders

Objectives

34.1 Identify pathophysiology of the following neurologic disorders: Alzheimer's disease, multiple sclerosis, Parkinson's disease, myasthenia gravis, amyotrophic lateral sclerosis, Huntington's disease, and Guillain-Barré syndrome.

34.2 Relate the signs and symptoms of the above listed disorders to the pathophysiology by recalling normal functioning of the neuroanatomy involved.

34.3 Discuss the profound physical and psychosocial adjustments required of clients (and their significant others) experiencing permanent or progressive neurologic problems.

34.4 Locate or develop standardized care plans for clients with the following common neurologic disorders: Alzheimer's disease, multiple sclerosis, Parkinson's disease, myasthenia gravis, amyotrophic lateral sclerosis, Huntington's disease, and Guillain-Barré syndrome.

34.5 Discuss the action, side effects, and nursing implications for medications given to treat Parkinsonism and myasthenia gravis.

Facilitating Student Learning

CLASSROOM

Class Assignments

- Ask students to prepare from their text a summary of the neurologic disorders, including definition, pathophysiology, usual signs and symptoms, diagnostic tests, and usual nursing care. Use this written assignment as a basis for class discussion.
- Assign groups of students to collect information on the financial hardships encountered by individuals with progressive neurologic disorders such as multiple sclerosis. Areas to consider include medical equipment rental, loss of income, hospital and medical costs, home environment alterations, home healthcare, and transportation adaptations. In class, ask the students to share their collected data.

Lecture/Discussion

- Supply students with case studies of clients in neurologic crises. Ask the students to identify the specific crisis, give emergency interventions and rationale for the interventions.

Guest Speaker

- Invite a physical therapist to discuss education for the client with Parkinson's disease. Ask the therapist to include the following topics: safety, maintaining joint mobility, and facial exercises.

CLINICAL

Clinical Site Activities

- Ask students to use the textbook summary of the neurologic disorder and compare the "textbook picture" with the clients to whom they have been assigned.
- Ask students to adapt the standardized plans they have located or developed to the clients to whom they have been assigned.
- Ask students to give the rationales for specific nursing interventions they have included in the nursing care plan for clients with neurologic disorders.
- Assign students to develop drug cards that include action, side effects, usual dosage, route of administration, and nursing implications for medications specific to neurologic disorders that their clients are receiving. If commercial drug cards are used, ask students to add rationale for use with their patients. Refer students to Tables 34–1, 34–2, and 34–3 in the text.
- Arrange clinical experiences with a home healthcare agency so students may provide home care of clients with neurologic disorders. Ask students to collect data that would reflect promotion of the person's independence in all aspects of care; i.e., decision-making, modification of home environment.
- Ask students to participate in interdisciplinary discharge planning conferences for clients with neurologic disorders in acute care settings.
- Ask students to collaborate with the primary nurse in completing discharge summary forms on clients with neurologic disorders.

Clinical Conference Activities

- Invite someone with a progressive neurologic disorder to share with the students the changes that were necessary in his or her life because of the disease's effects.
- Discuss the emotional impact of this illness. Refer students to the Bridges to Home Healthcare and Client Education Guides in the text.
- Obtain educational material from the various resources such as the Myasthenia Gravis Foundation to show as examples of information available to clients with the various degenerative neurologic disorders and their families. Refer students to Box 34–3 in the text.

CHAPTER

35

Nursing Care of Clients with Disorders of the Spinal Cord, Peripheral Nerves, and Cranial Nerves

OBJECTIVES

35.1 Compare the initial signs and symptoms of clients with spinal injuries at C3–C4, C5–C6, and L4–L5 levels.

35.2 Describe the signs and symptoms and the physiologic bases of autonomic dysreflexia (hyperreflexia).

35.3 Describe assessment findings with a ruptured lumbar and a cervical intervertebral disc.

35.4 Differentiate among the signs and symptoms resulting from injuries to the following peripheral nerves: radial, median, ulnar, sciatic, common peroneal, axillary, and long thoracic.

35.5 Describe clinical manifestations associated with the cranial nerve disorders trigeminal neuralgia and Bell's palsy.

35.6 Discuss emergency treatment for a victim of a suspected spinal cord injury.

35.7 List nursing interventions and their rationales for clients who are experiencing autonomic dysreflexia.

35.8 Identify nursing diagnoses and interventions for commonly occurring problems for clients with spinal cord injuries.

35.9 Explain, in general terms, medical-surgical interventions to stabilize cervical, thoracic, and lumbar spinal fractures.

35.10 Discuss the profound physical and psychosocial (including sexual) adjustments required of people, and their significant others, experiencing spinal cord injury.

35.11 Describe nursing care for the client having a laminectomy and spinal fusion.

Facilitating Student Learning

CLASSROOM

Class Assignment

- Assign students to complete the activities in the Study Guide for Chapter 35.

Lecture/Discussion

- Explain the results of injuries to one side of the spinal cord. Refer students to Figure 35–3 in the text.
- Using Table 35–3 in the text, lead class discussion on the rehabilitation potential for clients with spinal cord injuries at different cord levels. Include activities of daily living, work, sexuality, and environmental adaptations. Transparency 32–1(T) may be used.
- Discuss the impact on human sexuality resulting from a spinal cord injury and include how such an injury affects sexual functioning in males and females. Table 35–4 in the text may be used.
- Discuss nursing care for the client with a spinal cord injury. Chapter 35 of the text provides specific information organized by nursing diagnoses and collaborative problems.

Transparencies

- 44(M)—Level of Spinal Cord Injury
- 45(T)—Mechanisms of Spinal Injury
- 218(T)—Spine Immobilization Devices

Guest Speakers

- Invite a representative of the Spinal Cord Commission to participate in a discussion about services offered for clients with neurologic disorders.
- Invite members of the rehabilitation team to participate in a panel discussion of their contributions to the rehabilitation of the neurologically impaired client.

CLINICAL

Skills Laboratory

- Ask the students to use the restroom while in a wheelchair. Tell them to pretend their lower extremities are very weak and cannot take their full weight.
- Assign students to practice turning each other on the RotoRest bed and Stryker frame. Focus student attention on the safety precautions and the person's feelings of helplessness and fear associated with this equipment.

Clinical Site Activity

- Make arrangements for students to tour a rehabilitation institute if it is not possible to arrange a clinical rotation at that site.

Clinical Conference Activities

- Invite a person who has adapted to a neurologic disorder. Ask the guest to discuss his or her life changes from a physiologic and psychosocial point of view.
- Ask the students to imagine that they have a permanent cervical spinal cord injury and to share what changes they think this injury would have made in their activities during the past week.
- Develop communication guides for clients with spinal cord injuries who are at different stages of the grieving process. A member of the nursing psychiatric faculty may be invited to assist with the process. Once the communication guides are developed, ask the students to use them in a role play of an interaction.
- Invite an emergency medical technician to clinical conference to demonstrate emergency first aid for a victim of a suspected spinal cord injury.

Critical Points to Emphasize

SPINAL CORD INJURIES

- *Etiology*: most common cause is trauma
- *Flexion injury*: For example, head hits steering wheel or windshield and rupture of posterior ligaments results in forward dislocation of the vertebrae, may damage blood vessels leading to ischemia of cord
- *Hyperextension injury*: For example, chin hits object and head is thrown back, rupturing anterior ligament and fracturing posterior elements of vertebral body, may result in complete transsection of the cord
- *Compression injury*: person lands directly on head, sacrum, or feet after falling or jumping, force of impact fractures vertebrae and fragments compress cord, causing incomplete cord lesions
- *Pathophysiology*: most injuries occur at C1–2, C4–6, and T11–L2 as these are most mobile segments of the spine; microscopic bleeding at time of injury, edema within one hour of injury and peaking after 2–3 days and usually subsiding after 7 days, fragmentation of axonal covering and loss of myelin, tissue necrosis with macrophages engulfing debris leaving central cavity in injured spinal cord (called posttraumatic syringomyelia) as early as 9 days after injury, physiologic generalized stress response, automatic spinal reflex activity produces spasticity as recovery progresses
- *Clinical manifestations*: complete transsection results in immediate paralysis, paresthesia, bowel and bladder function below level of injury, hypotension and loss of temperature control (client assumes temperature of environment); incomplete injuries result in partial losses; a cervical injury results in quadriplegia, a thoracic or lumbar injury results in paraplegia, injuries above C4 may be fatal because of innervation of diaphragm
- *Autonomic hyperreflexia*: after spinal shock resolves, exaggerated sympathetic responses to noxious stimulus below level of injury produce hypertension, diaphoresis, piloerection, dilated pupils; baroreceptors stimulate parasympathetic nervous system in effort to decrease B/P resulting in bradycardia, flushing, and headache
- *Emergency Care*: assess baseline deficits; immobilize spine using spine board, hard neck collar, and safety straps around torso and legs; maintain patent airway and oxygenation; skeletal traction with skull tongs; cervical spine x-rays; normal saline IV; NG tube to suction; Foley catheter
- *Critical Care:* transfer to Stryker frame or RotoRest bed, continue with above treatment and add steroids, vasoactive medication as needed, suction prn to prevent aspiration, enteral or parenteral feedings as indicated to maintain nutrition if oral intake insufficient
- *Acute and Subacute Care*: establish functional goals, promote mobility (wheelchair, back brace) and prevent contractures, improve bladder and bowel control (Credé maneuver, catheterization methods, conditioned reflex activity), prevent pressure ulcers (AHCPR guidelines), reduce respiratory dysfunction (incentive spirometry), promote expression of sexuality (education and counseling), reduce pain (nonnarcotic analgesics and transcutaneous nerve stimulators), promote self-care, treat autonomic dysreflexia if it occurs (elevate head of bed to sitting position, check B/P, check for stimulus and remove, antihypertensive medication if necessary), prevent injury, help individual adjust to life changes (be realistic)

CHAPTER

36

Eye Disorders

OBJECTIVES

36.1 Demonstrate an accurate understanding of the structure, function, and vocabulary related to the human eye.

36.2 Describe assessment of clients with eye disorders.

36.3 Discuss the pathophysiology, treatment, and nursing care for clients with common disorders of the eye.

Facilitating Student Learning

CLASSROOM

Review Activities

- Assign students to review the structure and function of the eye.
- Assign students to review the cranial nerves related to vision.
- Review Chapter 11 for specific questions related to taking a ROS for the eye.
- Assign students to review vocabulary related to structure and function of the eye and eye disorders.

Lecture/Discussion

- Demonstrate a basic nursing assessment of the eye and related structures.
- Spend 15 minutes at the beginning of class reviewing the vocabulary on structure and function of the eye and eye disorders. This can be done using a "Jeopardy" format.
- Discuss the nurse's role in teaching health practices that will protect a person's vision.
- Discuss the incidence of vision impairment and the eye disorders that can result in damage to the eye.
- Discuss with students the effects of aging on the eye.
- Lead a discussion with students on the impact of loss of vision or changes in vision.
- Discuss the pathophysiologies associated with eye disorders.
- Discuss the medications commonly used with ophthalmic disorders, nursing implications, and patient teaching.
- Discuss medical and surgical interventions used with ophthalmic disorders.
- Discuss nursing care for persons having eye surgeries and care with other disorders of the eye.
- Discuss risks and preventive care for clients who are unable to close their eyelids.

Transparencies

- 46(T)—Anatomy of the Eye
- 47(T)—Correction of Common Refractive Errors

Group Activity

- Assign students to investigate and report on local and national rehabilitation resources for the blind and visually impaired.

CLINICAL

Skills Laboratory

- Pair students and assign them to take an ophthalmic history and do a physical examination of the eye.
- Question students during their practice examinations about which structure of the eye is being tested with the various procedures.
- Pair students and blindfold one of the pair. Ask the student who can see to orient his or her partner to a healthcare facility room; assist the person to walk in the halls; walk upstairs; and orient the person so they could eat a meal from a tray.

Clinical Site Activities

- Assign students to care for persons with ophthalmic disorders.
- Assign students to accompany persons to ophthalmic surgery and to plan and implement pre- and postoperative care.
- If it is not possible for the students to accompany a person in the healthcare facility to the OR, assign them to spend time in an outpatient surgical unit to observe ophthalmic surgery. Assign students to obtain a copy of the postoperative instructions given to persons having ophthalmic surgery and give rationale for the teaching items.
- Have students participate in discharge teaching for clients having eye surgery.

Clinical Conference Activity

- Ask students to share the experiences they had blindfolded in the Skills Laboratory assignment above. Bring into the discussion the significance of sight for people who have the sense intact and for those with the sense impaired.

Critical Points to Emphasize

OPEN ANGLE GLAUCOMA

- Most common type
- No early warning signs
- Diagnosed with tonometry
- Most common cause:
  —Decreased outflow of aqueous humor
- Clinical signs:
  —Increased intraocular pressure
  —Cupping or indentation of the optic nerve disc
  —Visual field defects
- Key medical interventions:
  —Miotics, beta-blockers, alpha adrenergics or carbonic anhydrase inhibitors
  —Surgical procedures with laser trabeculectomy, filtering procedures, or iridectomy
- Postop nursing interventions:
  —Teaching about eye protection, medications, not lying on operative side, signs of infections

CATARACT

- Pathophysiology of cataract development
- Signs and symptoms:
  —Blurred vision, monocular diplopia, photophobia, glare, and diminished or absent red reflex
- Surgical management:
  —Removal of opacified lens with or without lens implantation
- Complications:
  —Secondary glaucoma, infection, bleeding, macular edema, wound leaks
- Long-term complications:
  —Posterior capsule may become opacified
- Nursing Care:
  —Assessment, safety precautions postop, medication administration teaching, eye protection, activity, and pain management

CHAPTER

37

Ear Disorders

Objectives

37.1 Describe the structures and functions of the ear.

37.2 Identify elements of a complete assessment of the ear.

37.3 Discuss the pathophysiology and medical and nursing interventions for persons with disorders of the ear.

37.4 Differentiate among the types of hearing loss.

37.5 Discuss pathophysiologies and medical and nursing interventions for clients with balance disorders.

Facilitating Student Learning

CLASSROOM

Review Activity

- Assign students to review the structure and function of the ear and related structures.

Lecture/Discussion

- Demonstrate a basic nursing assessment of the ear, hearing, and equilibrium.
- Discuss the nurse's role in teaching health practices that protect the ears and hearing.
- Discuss disorders associated with the ears.
- Discuss medical and surgical interventions used to treat clients with disorders of the ears.
- Discuss nursing care for persons having ear surgery.
- Emphasize techniques which facilitate communication with persons who are hearing-impaired.
- Emphasize common medications that are ototoxic and nursing measures to assess for and prevent this complication.
- Discuss changes in hearing associated with aging.
- Emphasize safety concerns associated with caring for clients with balance disorders.

Transparencies

- 48(T)—Anatomy of the Ear
- 49(T)—Cochlear Implant to Restore Hearing

Group Activity

- Assign students to investigate and report on local and national rehabilitation resources for the hearing-impaired.

CLINICAL

Skills Laboratory

- Pair students and assign them to complete an assessment of the ear and related structures.

Clinical Site Activity

- Assign students to plan and implement care for persons who are hearing impaired and/or who have disorders of the ear or equilibrium.

Clinical Conference Activities

- Invite a person who is hearing-impaired to discuss ways of improving communication with persons whose main form of communication is sign language.
- Assign a group of students to obtain their healthcare facility's list of interpreters for sign language. If no list is available, assign students to develop a list of hospital employee interpreters and share the list with their clinical units.
- Work with students to develop a nursing care plan for a person with moderate hearing loss and a person with complete hearing loss.

Critical Points to Emphasize

HEARING IMPAIRMENT

- 80% of hearing impairments are caused by neural disorders
- Nation's #1 disability
- Common causes
- Differentiate between conductive and sensorineural hearing loss
- Signs of hearing loss
- Nursing roles in prevention of hearing loss
- Presence of tinnitus
- Medical diagnosis: H & P, audiometry
- Types and use of hearing aids and assistive listening devices
- Nursing care:
  —Assessment, communication strategies with hearing-impaired persons, assisting the client with coping, and teaching about hearing aids

VERTIGO

- Differentiate between vertigo and dizziness
- Cause of vertigo
- Types of disorders
- Pathophysiology
- Signs and symptoms
- Medical management: medications, vestibular rehabilitation
- Nursing management: assessment, safety considerations, assistance with changes in lifestyles, assistance with impaired communication, assessment for fluid and electrolyte imbalances

OTITIS MEDIA

- Infection of the middle ear
- Effects of chronic otitis
- Clinical manifestations: ear pain, changes in tympanic membrane, sensation of bubbling, crackles, or popping
- Serous otitis
- Medical Management:
  —Antibiotic therapy
  —C & S if drainage present
- Nursing interventions:
  —Teaching ways to open eustachian tubes, local heat, completing entire prescription of antibiotics
  —If disorder becomes chronic, a myringotomy may be performed
- Medical management: medications, vestibular rehabilitation
- Nursing management: assessment, safety considerations, assistance with changes in lifestyles, assistance with impaired communication, assessment for fluid and electrolyte imbalances

CHAPTER

38

Structure and Function of the Respiratory System

Objectives

38.1 Explain the structure and function of the upper and lower airways.

38.2 Explain the process of ventilation, perfusion, and gas exchange.

38.3 Describe the process of gas exchange that occurs in the alveolar-capillary system.

38.4 Describe the mechanical, neural, and chemical stimuli that can affect ventilation.

38.5 Discuss the defense mechanisms that protect the integrity of the respiratory system.

38.6 Describe the effects of aging on the lungs.

Facilitating Student Learning

CLASSROOM

Review Activity

- Give students a nongraded pretest on the basic concepts involved in ventilation, perfusion, and gas exchange.

Class Assignments

- Assign students to complete Chapter 38 in the Study Guide before class.
- Assign selected students to discuss in class one of the following: location and function of the respiratory center, one of the defense mechanisms that protect the integrity of the respiratory system, and the relationships among ventilation and perfusion, internal and external respiration, pulmonary blood flow, and gas transport.

Lecture/Discussion

- If the students have completed an anatomy and physiology course, this material should only be reviewed. Use the results from the pretest to determine which topics to include in the review.
- Use Transparencies 50(T) and 51(T) to clarify the structure of the respiratory system.
- Use an anatomical model to demonstrate structures of the lungs and conducting system.
- If you have access to multimedia, show a video or a CD-ROM of the respiratory system.
- Review the concepts of ventilation, perfusion, and gas exchange.
- Review osmosis, diffusion, and active transport as they apply to gas transport.

Transparencies

- 50(T)—The Upper Respiratory Tract
- 51(T)—The Lower Respiratory Tract
- Figure 38-9—Gas Exchange
- Figure 38-8—The Respiratory Membrane
- Figure 38-10—Normal Inspiration and Expiration
- Figure 38-12—Partial Pressures of Gases During Normal Respirations

Group Activities

- Divide the class into small groups. Ask each group to discuss the factors necessary for normal respiration.
- Divide the class into small groups. Ask each group to discuss mechanical and chemical stimuli that can affect ventilation.

CHAPTER

39

Assessment of Clients with Respiratory Disorders

Objectives

39.1 Give rationale for a focused respiratory assessment, including history-taking and physical examination.

39.2 Perform a basic respiratory health history and physical examination.

39.3 Prepare clients and significant others, both physically and psychologically, for various diagnostic procedures.

39.4 Discuss nursing responsibilities related to selected diagnostic procedures used to evaluate respiratory function.

Facilitating Student Learning

CLASSROOM

Class Assignments

- Assign students to listen to simulated normal and abnormal lung sounds. Ask them to compare these sounds to the information in Tables 39-2 and 39-3.
- Ask selected students to discuss common noninvasive methods of monitoring the respiratory status: oximetry, capnography, transcutaneous measurements of PO_2.
- Ask students to discuss pulmonary function test indicators (Table 36-4).

Lecture/Discussion

- Focus a lecture on pertinent aspects of the respiratory history. Discuss with students general questions to be included in an initial respiratory history and the elements of an extensive respiratory history.
- Use your school's data format and framework as a lecture guide. The Appendix of the Study Guide has a functional health pattern blank grid that can be copied.
- Focus the lecture on pertinent aspects of basic respiratory physical examination; i.e., abnormalities found during respiratory examination and indicators of respiratory dysfunction.
- Emphasize the concept of noninvasive and invasive tests and the general assumptions that can be made; i.e., usually a noninvasive test does not require an informed consent and involves minimal risks, teaching, and preparation.
- Ask students to discuss nursing responsibilities associated with the various diagnostic procedures presented in this chapter. Focus on preprocedure, during the procedure, and postprocedure care.

Transparencies

- 50(T)—The Upper Respiratory Tract
- 51(T)—The Lower Respiratory Tract
- 52(T)—Respiratory Examination: Posterior (Figure 39-2)
- 53(T)—Respiratory Examination: Lateral (Figure 39-2)
- 54(T)—Respiratory Examination: Anterior
- 55(T)—Chest Deformities (Figure 36-3)
- 56(T)—Location of Normal Breath Sounds: Anterior (Figure 39-8)
- 57(T)—Location of Normal Breath Sounds: Posterior (Figure 39-8)
- 58(T)—Oxyhemoglobin Dissociation Curve (Figure 58)
- Normal Physical Assessment Findings (Example Page 1042)
- Clubbing (Figure 39-4)
- Sequence of Palpation, Percussion, and Auscultation (Figure 39-6)

Guest Speaker

- Invite a pulmonary function technician to class to discuss pulmonary function tests. Ask the technician to discuss the following: purposes and limitations of the tests and factors that are measured during the tests.

Group Activities

- Role play the collection of a respiratory history.
- Divide the class into small groups and provide each group with a case study of an individual with a respiratory disorder. Ask the groups to analyze the assessed data for evidence of common respiratory symptoms (cough, sputum production, dyspnea, hemoptysis, chest pain, and wheezing). Ask them to discuss what additional assessment data related to these symptoms need to be collected.

- Divide the class into small groups and provide each group a list of arterial blood gas values. Ask students to determine which values are abnormal and to discuss interpretation of the findings. In addition, ask the students to discuss therapeutic interventions that could be used to improve or correct those that are abnormal.
- Ask small groups of students to explore how each of the following radiographic and/or sonographic procedures is used to evaluate the respiratory status of an individual. In addition, ask students to discuss the procedure and the pre- and postprocedure care of the client.

  —chest x-ray —bronchography

  —tomograms —pulmonary angiography

  —CAT scan —ultrasonography
- Discuss procedure for obtaining a sputum specimen. Role play and have students practice obtaining a sputum specimen. Allow time for the students to share their thoughts and feelings on the ease or difficulty of giving a sputum specimen. Guide students in applying the problems encountered to an ill client. Discuss direct and indirect methods of obtaining a specimen, and indications for each.

CLINICAL

Skills Laboratory

- Using inspection, percussion, palpation, and auscultation, demonstrate a respiratory physical examination. Use Transparencies 56(T) and 57(T) to clarify sequence for thoracic percussion and auscultation.
- Demonstrate technique for obtaining an arterial blood gas sample. Be certain to demonstrate the Allen's test for assessing collateral circulation in the hand.
- Demonstrate thoracentesis procedure. Include with the demonstration an explanation of the pre- and postprocedure care of the individual.
- Simulate parts of pulmonary function tests by using an incentive spirometer. If your school permits, use the CPR mouth covers over the mouthpiece and let students practice this exercise.

Clinical Site Activities

- Assign students to obtain a health history from a client diagnosed as having a respiratory disorder. If a client with a respiratory disorder is not available, assessment of the respiratory history of any client would be valuable.
- Ask students to perform a basic respiratory physical examination on assigned individual.
- Suggest students listen to breath sounds on all of their clients. Students can check the physician's progress notes for verification of abnormal breath sounds. Also, have them read chest x-ray reports or other diagnostic reports to compare and analyze their findings.
- Assign students to observe pulmonary function tests. Ask students to describe the preparation of the client, the specific test conducted, and factors measured by the test.
- Assign students to accompany a respiratory therapist. This is a valuable experience, so allow time for the students to share their experience either verbally or in writing. Often, they will identify safe and unsafe techniques as well as a variety of assessment findings. The experience can also be used to emphasize evaluation of medications and interventions, such as coughing, deep breathing, suctioning, and chest physiotherapy.
- Arrange for students to observe a bronchoscopy. Ask students to note not only the procedure but the reactions of the client.

Clinical Conference Activities

- Ask students to share their assessment data and to identify significant findings.
- Ask students to be prepared to discuss how diagnostic data on the assigned client were interpreted to determine the individual's respiratory status.
- Ask students to discuss diagnostic testing observations (See Clinical Site Activities).

CHAPTER

40

Nursing Care of Clients with Upper Airway Disorders

Objectives

40.1 Discuss etiology, incidence, risk factors, clinical manifestations, complications, diagnostic tests, and medical-surgical treatment of selected disorders of the upper airway.

40.2 Describe nursing management of the client with selected disorders of the upper airway.

40.3 Discuss respiratory disorders that produce chronic airway obstruction.

40.4 Plan care for a client with a tracheostomy.

Facilitating Student Learning

CLASSROOM

Review Activities

- Assign students to review the structures and functions of the upper airway.
- Assign students to review tracheostomy care and suctioning procedure in a basic skills book. If necessary, request that they go to the psychomotor skills laboratory to practice the technique.

Class Assignments

- Assign students to complete Chapter 40 of the Study Guide before class.
- Provide students with a case study of a client scheduled for a total laryngectomy. Ask students to identify appropriate nursing diagnoses and interventions.
- Assign students to develop learning/teaching guidelines for a client with a laryngectomy. Ask them to include information on communication methods, airway care, wound and skin care, personal hygiene, safety, and health promotion measures.
- Using the guidelines developed by the students, use role playing to demonstrate teaching the information.
- Assign selected students to assess community resources available to the individual with a laryngectomy, such as the American Cancer Society, Laryngectomy Club, Lost Cord Club, and Nu Voice Club. Have them share their information with the class.

Lecture/Discussion

- Focus on laryngeal disorders. Spend most of the class time discussing medical/surgical management of laryngeal cancer. Other content in the chapter can be handled by allowing time in class for questions regarding the Study Guide material.
- Emphasize the common assessment findings associated with laryngeal disorders. Identify aspects to be assessed during the nursing health history.
- Focus on the client requiring a partial laryngectomy, total laryngectomy, and/or radical neck dissection.
- Differentiate among the different surgical approaches. Use Transparency 60(T) to clarify airway structure and function before and after a total laryngectomy. Include a discussion of possible complications after laryngeal surgery and the functional alterations due to total laryngectomy. Use Transparency 61(T) to clarify tracheoesophageal puncture method of voice rehabilitation.
- Ask students to discuss the preoperative and postoperative care of a client requiring surgery for laryngeal disorders.

Transparencies

- 60(T)—Airflow Through the Nose and Mouth. A, Normal, B, with Tracheostomy
- 61(T)—Tracheoesophageal Puncture
- 62(T)—Tracheostomy Dressings

Guest Speakers

- Invite someone from a Laryngectomy Club, Lost Cord Club, or Nu Voice Club to class to talk to the students. Ask him or her to discuss communication methods available to the person with a laryngectomy.
- Invite a speech therapist to discuss esophageal speech. Ask the therapist to discuss physiologic and psychosocial factors that promote successful speech rehabilitation.

CLINICAL

Skills Laboratory

- Role play preparation of the client for a partial laryngectomy.
- Review care of the client with a tracheostomy tube.

- Display various types of tracheostomy tubes for students to review.
- Role play preparation of the client for a total laryngectomy.
- Role play discharge teaching for the client with a total laryngectomy.

Clinical Site Activities

- Many of the disorders of the upper respiratory tract are treated on an outpatient basis. It may not be possible to assign students to clients with these disorders. You can arrange for the students to have an observational experience in an ear, nose, and throat clinic. At the clinic, assign students to assess a client with an upper airway disorder.
- Assign students to care for a client scheduled for a tonsillectomy. (This assignment will be easier to achieve during a nursing of children rotation.)
- Assign students to an oncology unit or an ear, nose, and throat unit. Clients with laryngeal disorders should be assigned if possible.
- Assign students to an observational experience in a speech rehabilitation department.

Clinical Conference Activities

- Ask students to share their clinical experiences.
- Ask students to share their assessment findings for their clients. Have the clinical conference group discuss the significance of the findings. Emphasize findings that correlate with upper airway disorders.
- Invite a nutritionist to discuss the nutritional needs of a client having laryngectomy surgery. Ask the nutritionist to include ways of adapting the person's dietary intake to meet these needs.

CHAPTER

41

Nursing Care of Clients with Disorders of the Lower Airways and Pulmonary Vessels

Objectives

41.1 Describe the incidence, etiology, risk factors, clinical manifestations, diagnostic tests, and complications associated with disorders of the lower airways and pulmonary vessels.

41.2 Summarize the medical/surgical management of selected disorders of the lower airways and pulmonary vessels.

41.3 Discuss the nursing management of disorders of the lower airways and pulmonary vessels.

41.4 Discuss the physical and psychosocial adjustments required of clients with chronic lower respiratory disorders.

Facilitating Student Learning

CLASSROOM

Review Activities

- Assign students to review the structure and function of the lower airway.
- Ask students to review blood gas analysis and the significance of abnormal findings.

Class Assignments

- Assign students to complete Chapter 41 in the Study Guide before class.
- Have students select a lower airway disorder that they want to study in more depth. Assign students to find two journal articles that address this disorder (one of the articles should be a nursing research study). Ask the students to share findings with the class.
- Assign students to develop drug cards for selected medications.
- Assign selected students to discuss lung volume reduction surgery and lung transplant.
- Provide the students with a list of arterial blood gas values. Ask the students to interpret these values and relate their interpretations to respiratory function for clients with chronic obstructive pulmonary disease (COPD), asthma, and pulmonary embolus.

Lecture/Discussion

- This chapter contains information on many important disorders. Review your curriculum to determine if any of these disorders are discussed in other courses. Emphasize asthma, COPD, and pulmonary embolus. Other disorders can be covered through the Study Guide or separate study sheets.
- Focus a lecture on asthma. Emphasize the two types of asthma: intrinsic and extrinsic. Discuss the pathogenesis of each type, clarifying the parasympathetic and sympathetic response seen in intrinsic asthma and the hypersensitivity reaction associated with extrinsic asthma. Focus on prevention of episodes and treatment of acute episodes. Nursing management of the client with asthma can be covered in a discussion format. Provide students with a case study and have the students determine the nursing care required by the client in the study.
- Focus a lecture on COPD. Use pulmonary emphysema as the model for this group of conditions. Discuss the etiology, pathophysiology, clinical manifestations, diagnostic tests, complications, and medical treatment associated with pulmonary emphysema. Use Transparencies 63(T)–67(T) to clarify content. Ask students to discuss nursing interventions for clients with emphysema.
- Focus a lecture on pulmonary embolus. Discuss the etiology, pathophysiology, clinical manifestations, diagnostic tests, complications, and medical treatment. Ask students to discuss nursing interventions for clients with pulmonary embolus.

Transparencies

- 63(T)—Types of Emphysema (Figure 41-3)
- 64(T)—Types of Emphysema: Centriacinar
- 65(T)—Types of Emphysema: Panacinar
- 66(T)—Clinical Manifestations of COPD (Figure 41-4)
- 67(T)—Chest Wall Changes Associated with COPD (Figure 41-7)
- Table 41-1—Action Plan for Adult Asthma
- Table 41-2—ABGs with Asthma
- Tables 41-1–41-3—Clinical Manifestations of Asthma, Bronchitis, COPD

Guest Speakers

- Invite a nutritionist to class to discuss the dietary needs of the client with COPD.
- Invite a community health nurse to class to discuss the post-hospital care of a client in the community.

Group Activities

- Divide the class into small groups and provide each group with a case study of an individual with chronic bronchitis and an individual with emphysema. Ask students to compare and contrast the assessment findings for these two conditions and to discuss the pathophysiologic bases for these findings.
- Divide the class into three groups. Provide each group with a case study of a client with chronic bronchitis, emphysema, or asthma. Ask students to develop comprehensive care plans for the client. After the plans are completed, ask each group to share with the whole class.

CLINICAL

Skills Laboratory

- Use role playing to demonstrate teaching needs of a client with emphysema.

Clinical Site Activities

- Assign students to care for a client with a lower airway disorder. Clients with asthma, bronchitis, and emphysema are frequently hospitalized for evaluation and stabilization of their disease. Ask students to complete an assessment of the assigned client.
- Ask students to provide the pathophysiologic bases for the assessed data.
- Ask students to develop a comprehensive care plan based on the assessed data. Have them consider teaching and post-hospital care needs.
- Have students develop drug cards for selected medications used to treat lower airway disorders.

Clinical Conference Activities

- Ask students to share their assessment findings. Have the conference group discuss the significance of these findings.
- Have students identify the diagnostic procedures used to confirm the medical diagnosis of the assigned client.
- Ask students to share their observation experiences (see Clinical Site Activities). Assign students to identify two nursing diagnoses and four nursing interventions for each diagnosis that are appropriate for the client observed.
- Invite a dietitian to conference to discuss the nutritional needs of clients with lower respiratory disorders. Ask the dietitian to discuss how meals can be adapted to meet the needs of clients with COPD, chronic bronchitis, or restrictive lung disease.
- Invite a person with asthma and/or COPD to discuss what it is like to have a chronic respiratory illness.

CHAPTER

42

Nursing Care of Clients with Disorders of the Lung Parenchyma and Pleura

Objectives

42.1 Describe the incidence, etiology, risk factors, clinical manifestations, diagnostic tests, and complications associated with disorders of the lung parenchyma and pleura.

42.2 Summarize the medical and surgical management of selected disorders of the lung parenchyma and pleura.

42.3 Discuss the nursing management of disorders of the lung parenchyma and pleura.

42.4 Discuss the nursing management of clients with chest tubes or being mechanically ventilated.

Facilitating Student Learning

CLASSROOM

Review Activities

- Assign students to review the structure and function of the lower airway.
- Ask students to review blood gas analysis and the significance of abnormal findings.
- Ask students to think about blood gas analysis. Are the readings similar or different for disorders of the upper airway, lower airway, and lung parenchyma and pleura?

Class Assignments

- Assign students to complete Chapter 42 in the Study Guide before class.
- Have students select a disorder of the lung parenchyma or pleura that they want to study in more depth. Assign students to find two journal articles that address this disorder (one of the articles should be a nursing research study). Ask the students to share findings with the class.
- Assign students to develop drug cards for selected tuberculosis medications, chemotherapeutic agents used in lung cancer, and medications to treat adult respiratory distress syndrome (ARDS).
- Assign selected students to discuss the following thoracic surgical procedures: exploratory thoracotomy, resection pulmonary surgery, decortication, and thoracoplasty.
- Provide the students with a list of arterial blood gas values. Ask the students to interpret these values and relate their interpretations to respiratory function and complications of chest surgery.

Lecture/Discussion

- This chapter contains information on many important disorders. Review your curriculum to determine if any of these disorders are discussed in other courses. Emphasize pneumonia, pulmonary tuberculosis, adult respiratory distress syndrome, malignant lung tumors, and cystic fibrosis. Other disorders can be covered through the Study Guide or separate study sheets.
- Focus a lecture on pneumonia. Use pneumococcal pneumonia as the model for bacterial pneumonia. Discuss the etiology, pathophysiology, clinical manifestations, diagnostic tests, complications, and medical treatment associated with pneumonia. A case study of an elderly client with pneumococcal pneumonia would facilitate discussion of this disorder. Have students identify appropriate nursing diagnoses for this client and to determine expected outcomes that would evaluate the effectiveness of their care.
- Focus a lecture on pulmonary tuberculosis; extrapulmonary tuberculosis can be presented as a complication of pulmonary TB instead of a separate disorder. Emphasize that the number of reported cases of TB is increasing. Include discussion of the risk factors and pathophysiology of the primary infection. Have students provide the clinical manifestations and medical and nursing management of clients with pulmonary TB.
- If cystic fibrosis is not discussed in pediatric courses, focus a lecture on cystic fibrosis. Emphasize the adult aspect of the disorder. Focus on the adult with cystic fibrosis and the developmental and psychosocial problems and issues. Review the etiology and pathophysiology if needed.
- Focus a lecture on ARDS. Emphasize the pathophysiology of ARDS and the clinical disorders that may trigger the condition. Use Transparency 68(T) to clarify pathophysiology.

- Focus a lecture on malignant lung neoplasms. Emphasize the risk factors, pathology, clinical manifestations, diagnostic tests, complications, and medical management for these disorders. Discuss preoperative and postoperative assessment and intervention for the client having chest surgery. Discuss potential complications following chest surgery. Assist students to identify appropriate nursing diagnoses and interventions. Use Transparency 69(T) to clarify splinting techniques.
- Review purposes of and factors affecting closed chest drainage. Review the principles used in all closed drainage systems. Discuss these principles as they relate to several types of closed chest drainage systems.
- Review nursing assessment and interventions associated with water-seal drainage. Ask students to recall appropriate nursing measures if any accidents or problems involving closed chest drainage occur.
- Focus a lecture on nursing care of a client on mechanical ventilation.

Transparencies

- 68(T)—Pathophysiology of ARDS
- 69(T)—Splinting Techniques (Figure 42-6)
- 72(T)—Pulmonary Resections (Figure 42-5)
- Figure 42-7—Arm and Shoulder Exercises
- Figure 42-8—Chest Drainage System
- Understanding ARDS and Its Treatment Algorithm

Guest Speakers

- Invite a nutritionist to class to discuss the dietary needs of clients with pneumonia, tuberculosis, and lung cancer.
- Invite a community health nurse to class to discuss the post-hospital care of the client in the community.
- Ask a nurse from the local public health department to discuss pulmonary tuberculosis. Ask the person to include information on pathology, primary and secondary TB disease, assessment findings, and nursing and medical intervention.
- Invite a clinical nurse specialist to discuss the nursing care of a client following chest surgery. Ask the nurse to discuss assessment measures, nursing diagnoses, and interventions appropriate for this individual.

Group Activity

- Divide the class into small groups and provide each group a case study of a client with a complication of chest surgery. Ask the students to identify the complication and to develop a plan of care that addresses the needs of the client.

CLINICAL

Skills Laboratory

- Use role playing to demonstrate teaching needs of a client scheduled for chest surgery.
- Demonstrate techniques for splinting the chest.
- Demonstrate postoperative exercises following chest surgery.
- For review purposes, set up the following types of closed chest drainage systems: one-bottle, two-bottle, and three-bottle water-seal apparatus, two-bottle water-seal apparatus with suction, and Pleur-evac.
- Review and practice tracheostomy and endotracheal suctioning.

Clinical Site Activities

- Assign students to care for a client with lung cancer. Clients with lung cancer frequently have pneumonia and pleural effusions at some point during their illnesses. Ask students to complete an assessment of the assigned client.
- Ask students to provide the pathophysiologic bases for the assessed data.
- Ask students to develop a comprehensive care plan based on the assessed data. Have them consider teaching and post-hospital care needs.
- Have students develop drug cards for selected medications used to treat lower airway disorders.
- Assign students to a respiratory care unit to observe the care of a client after chest surgery.
- Assign students to a critical care unit to care for a client on mechanical ventilation.
- Arrange for students to observe thoracic surgery and the immediate postoperative care of the client in the recovery room.

Clinical Conference Activities

- Ask students to share their clients' assessment findings. Have the conference group discuss the significance of these findings.
- Have students identify the diagnostic procedures used to confirm the medical diagnosis of their assigned client.
- Ask students to share their observation experiences (see Clinical Site Activities). Assign students to identify two nursing diagnoses and four nursing interventions for each diagnosis that are appropriate for the client observed.
- Invite a dietitian to conference to discuss the nutritional needs of clients with disorders of the lung parenchyma and pleura. Ask the dietitian to discuss how meals can be adapted to meet the needs of these clients.
- Invite a clinical nurse specialist or critical care nurse to conference to discuss mechanical ventilators and the associated nursing care and responsibilities.

CHAPTER

43

Structure and Function of the Heart

Objectives

43.1 Discuss normal cardiac structure and function.

43.2 State the two primary functions of the heart.

43.3 Diagram normal blood flow through the heart chambers and valves.

43.4 Explain the factors that influence the mechanical properties of the heart, including preload, afterload, and contractile state.

43.5 List factors that will cause variations in heart rate.

43.6 Discuss the effects of aging on the cardiovascular system.

Facilitating Student Learning

CLASSROOM

Review Activities

- Ask students to review notes and/or textbook from a previous anatomy and physiology course.
- Ask students to complete Chapter 43 of the Study Guide before class.

Class Assignments

- Assign selected students to discuss in class one of the following: electrophysiology of the heart, hemodynamics of blood flow, and generation of normal heart sounds.
- Assign students to monitor the pulse and blood pressure of two individuals in different age groups. Ask students to discuss in class the values obtained and explain the reasons for the differences.

Lecture/Discussion

- Review the normal anatomy and physiology of the cardiovascular (CV) system.
- Use transparencies to clarify the circulation of blood through the heart, coronary artery blood flow, and the conduction system of the heart.
- Use an anatomical heart model to clarify structure of the heart. Use a model that allows both the external and internal structures to be seen.

Transparencies

- 73(T)—Chambers of the Heart
- 74(T)—Blood Supply to the Myocardium
- 75(T)—Major Systemic Arteries
- 76(T)—Major Systemic Veins
- Figure 43-1—Systemic Circulation
- Figure 43-4—The Valves of the Heart
- Figure 43-13—Factors Affecting Blood Pressure

Group Activities

- Divide students into small groups, and ask each group to explore how two or three of the following factors affect the rate, rhythm, and/or volume of the pulse. Later, bring the groups together and have the students share their findings with the entire class. Ask the groups to provide the rationale for their findings.
  1. Decreased elasticity of arterial wall
  2. Fear
  3. Running
  4. Increased metabolism
  5. Old age
  6. Decreased metabolism
  7. Infancy
  8. Obesity
  9. Gender
  10. Decreased blood volume
- Ask small groups of students to explore how several of the following factors affect blood pressure. Ask them to share their answers with the class and to give the rationale for their answers.
  1. Increased or decreased arterial blood volume
  2. Age
  3. Position (sitting, lying, standing)
  4. Metabolic rate
  5. Increased peripheral resistance
  6. Increased or decreased cardiac output
  7. Increased or decreased metabolism

CHAPTER

44

Assessment of Clients with Cardiac Disorders

OBJECTIVES

44.1 Obtain a health history that focuses on the client's cardiovascular (CV) status.

44.2 Perform a basic CV physical examination.

44.3 Prepare the client both physically and psychologically for diagnostic studies.

44.4 Describe nursing responsibilities for selected diagnostic procedures used to evaluate CV function.

Facilitating Student Learning

CLASSROOM

Class Assignments

- Assign students to complete Chapter 44 in the Study Guide before class.
- Assign students to listen to simulated normal and abnormal heart sounds on a heart sound simulator.
- Assign students to interview their family members to determine their existing CV risk factors.
- Ask students to bring a newspaper or nonprofessional magazine article on the subject of CV risk factors. Discuss these articles in class, focusing on the quality of information being distributed to the public.

Lecture/Discussion

- Focus discussion on pertinent aspects of CV history; i.e., major symptoms of CV disorders and presence of risk factors.
- Role play collecting a health history from a client with a CV disorder.
- Focus discussion on pertinent aspects of basic CV physical examination; i.e., general appearance, blood pressure, pulse, and heart and lung sounds.
- Have students use Chapter 44 as a reference, but do not have them remember every aspect of each diagnostic study. Instead, focus on several of the more commonly seen diagnostic studies.
- Focus discussion on nursing responsibilities associated with various diagnostic procedures.

Transparencies

- 77(T)—Precordial Locations for Cardiac Palpation and Auscultation of Heart Sounds
- Figure 44–5—Relationship of Heart Sounds to Events During Cardiac Cycle

Group Activities

- Divide students into small groups, and provide each group with a case study including CV history, physical examination findings, and results from diagnostic studies. Ask students to evaluate the data and draw conclusions about the individual's CV status.
- Divide students into small groups, and ask each group to explore how each of the following conditions affects cardiac output. Discuss their answers in class.
  1. Old age
  2. Exercise
  3. Oral fluid intake
  4. Acute congestive heart failure
  5. Shock
  6. Heat stroke
  7. Pregnancy
  8. Valvular heart disease
- Ask small groups of students to explore how each of the following laboratory tests is used to evaluate the cardiac status of an individual.
  1. Leukocyte count
  2. Creatine kinase
  3. Lactic acid dehydrogenase
  4. Serum potassium
  5. Blood urea nitrogen
  6. Erythrocyte count
  7. Serum calcium
  8. Serum lipids

CLINICAL

Skills Laboratory

- Demonstrate assessment skills appropriate for students at this level: assessment of jugular vein distention, examination of carotid arteries, and auscultation of heart sounds. Transparency 77(T) could be used for clarification of material.
- Demonstrate appropriate diagnostic equipment and procedures: central venous pressure setup, PA flow-directed catheter (Swan-Ganz catheter), and electrocardiogram techniques. Figures 44–4 and 44–9 will help clarify placement of ECG electrodes and normal ECG pattern.

Clinical Site Activities

- Assign students to obtain a health history from a client diagnosed as having a CV disorder; e.g., hypertension, angina, or mitral valve prolapse.
- Ask students to perform a basic CV physical examination on an assigned client.
- Suggest that students auscultate heart sounds on every client assigned to them. If students detect abnormal heart sounds, they should refer to the physician's physical examination report in the client's chart for validation of their findings.
- Assign students to observe at least one major diagnostic test; e.g., echocardiogram, angiogram, cardiac catheterization, myocardial imaging, or stress testing.

Clinical Conference Activities

- Ask students to be prepared to discuss how diagnostic data on the assigned client were interpreted to determine the client's CV status.
- Ask students to discuss diagnostic testing observations. (See Clinical Site Activities.)

CHAPTER

45

Nursing Care of Clients with Disorders of Cardiac Function

Objectives

45.1 Describe the pathogenesis of atherosclerosis.

45.2 Discuss risk factors associated with coronary artery disease.

45.3 Describe the etiology and clinical manifestations of the following cardiac disorders: angina pectoris, myocardial infarction, and congestive heart failure.

45.4 Describe diagnostic studies used to assess clients with angina pectoris, myocardial infarction, and congestive heart failure.

45.5 Describe medical management and nursing management for clients with cardiac disorders.

45.6 Explain rationale for selected nursing interventions.

Facilitating Student Learning

CLASSROOM

Review Activities

- Assign students to review normal anatomy and physiology of the cardiovascular system.
- Ask students to go to the Psychomotor Skills Laboratory and review ECG monitoring.
- Ask students to review appropriate sections of Chapter 44.
- Assign students to complete Chapter 45 in the Study Guide before class.

Class Assignments

- Ask students to assess a family member for risk factors of coronary artery disease (CAD).
- Use role playing to demonstrate teaching the client with angina pectoris. Have students include dietary restrictions, methods to prevent and/or control episodes, and instructions for taking nitroglycerin.
- Use role playing to demonstrate assessment of an individual with a myocardial infarction (MI). Provide the student who portrays the client a brief cardiac history. Ask class members to write nursing diagnoses, goals, and interventions based on the assessed data collected by the nurse.
- Ask students to discuss the pathophysiologic bases for the assessed data collected during role playing.
- Assign selected students to discuss medical management of a client with an acute MI. Ask the class to discuss rationales for the therapy and related nursing responsibilities.
- Supply students with a case study of a client with heart failure. Ask the students to identify the subjective and objective manifestations and the form of congestive heart failure depicted in the case study.
- Ask students to explain how the following conditions might precipitate heart failure:
  1. Anemia
  2. Infections
  3. Hypervolemia
  4. Pregnancy
  5. Pulmonary disease
  6. Physical or emotional stress
- Ask the students to explain why the nurse's observations and assessments are important in the care of a client with cardiac dysrhythmia.
- Present a case study of a client with a cardiac dysrhythmia secondary to MI. Ask the students to develop nursing diagnoses, expected outcomes, and nursing interventions based on the assessed data.
- Ask the students to rank the following interventions in order of priority for clients experiencing an acute MI and give the rationale for each intervention.

  _____ Start oxygen

  _____ Draw blood for cardiac enzymes

  _____ Start two IVs

  _____ Start a heparin infusion

  _____ Relieve chest pain

  _____ Obtain chest x-ray

  _____ Obtain admission history and physical examination findings

  _____ Place the client on a continuous ECG monitor

  _____ Administer stool softener and aspirin

  _____ Administer nitroglycerin intravenous infusion

  _____ Obtain history data pertinent for thrombolytic therapy

  _____ Orient the client to room and CCU routines

- Present a case study of a client with a temporary or permanent pacemaker. Ask the students to develop nursing diagnoses, expected outcomes, and nursing interventions based on the assessed data.
- Use the CareMap for a pacemaker in Appendix D. Give the students baseline data for each problem, additional data for after the insertion, and discharge teaching. Have the students evaluate the client's progress toward meeting the goals.

Lecture/Discussion

- This chapter contains many important concepts. Allow sufficient time for coverage of the material and assimilation of the content.
- Focus initial presentation on the pathogenesis of atherosclerosis. Because this is the basis for many cardiac disorders, it is important that students have a clear understanding of this concept.
- Obtain specimens of animal arteries affected by atherosclerosis to show to the class.
- Discuss the relationship between atherosclerosis and myocardial ischemia and the relationship between myocardial ischemia and metabolic needs. Present the metabolic demands of various activities. Ask the students to explain how nurses can intervene to decrease metabolic requirements.
- Stress morphologic changes that follow an MI. Correlate these with the changes seen in isoenzyme, leukocyte, CPK-MB, and LDH levels.
- Discuss the pathophysiology of heart failure. Emphasize that understanding this aspect will facilitate the application of the nursing process.
- Stress the normal compensatory mechanisms of the heart.
- Discuss nursing measures specific for a client with heart failure. Have students supply the rationales for these measures.
- Give a lecture on the pathophysiology of cardiac dysrhythmias.
- Clarify classification of dysrhythmias. Emphasize the classification system based on where the dysrhythmia originates in the heart.
- Discuss nursing measures specific for a client with cardiac dysrhythmias. Stress assessment skills needed to evaluate cardiac rhythms.
- Discuss nursing management of the client after coronary artery bypass grafting (CABG) and percutaneous transluminal coronary angioplasty (PTCA).
- Refer to Appendix D5, Coordinated CareMaps for CABG/PTCA as a guide for care planning.

Transparencies

- 80(T)—Cross-Section of Artery (Figure 42–1)
- 81(T)—Areas of Myocardium Affected by Arterial Insufficiency
- Box 45–1—Risk Factor for CAD
- Figure 45–2—Response to Injury Theory of Atherogenesis
- Figure 45–3—PTCA
- Figure 45–4—Atherectomy
- Figure 45–5—Placement of a Coronary Stint
- Figure 45–6—Coronary Artery Bypass Graft
- Box 45–2—Factors Influencing Myocardial Supply and Demand
- Flowchart—Understanding Myocardial Infarction and Its Treatment
- Figure 45–7—Depth of Infarction
- Figure 45–11—Laboratory Tests

Guest Speakers

- Invite a CV rehabilitation nurse to discuss the usual program prescribed for a client recuperating from an MI.
- Invite a CV clinical specialist to discuss nursing diagnoses and nursing interventions commonly seen with individuals in congestive heart failure.

CLINICAL

Skills Laboratory

- Demonstrate cardiopulmonary resuscitation (CPR) techniques.
- Require that each student obtain cardiopulmonary life support credentials.

Clinical Site Activities

- Assign students to assess a client who has CAD. (This may not be the client's primary medical diagnosis.)
- Ask students to evaluate the ECG tracing from the record of assigned client.
- Ask students to check the chart of the assigned client for cholesterol and lipoprotein levels and to explain the significance of their findings.
- Ask students to develop a plan of care that addresses the risk factors apparent in the client.
- If you are not able to assign students to a client with angina pectoris, MI, or cardiac dysrhythmias, you might consider the following activities:
  - —Ask students to develop a discharge plan for a client recuperating from an MI. They should consider the following: drugs, dietary restrictions, exercise, and activities (including sexual activities).
  - —Assign each student to observe in the coronary care unit (AMCU, CCU, or postcoronary surgical unit).
  - —Assign each student to observe in a cardiac rehabilitation unit.
- Assign students to assess a client for precipitating causes of congestive heart failure.
- Assign students to assess a client who has heart failure as a primary or secondary medical diagnosis. (Elderly clients frequently have congestive heart failure as a secondary medical diagnosis.)
- Ask students to develop a care plan that includes one nursing diagnosis commonly seen in clients with heart failure.
- Ask students to give rationales for specific nursing interventions included in the care plan.
- Ask students to develop a discharge plan for a client with congestive heart failure that considers fluid and sodium intake, drugs, exercise, and activities.
- Assign students to locate the emergency equipment on the unit and explore the crash cart.
- Assign students to observe scheduled cardioversions and pacemaker insertions.
- Assign students to observe an autopsy. Each student should identify areas of the body where atherosclerosis was detected and explain the significance of these findings.
- Assign students to develop drug cards that include pharmacologic action, expected physiologic response, side effects, usual dosage, route of administration, and nursing implications for selected vasodilators, beta-adrenergic blocking agents, inotropic agents, antiarrhythmic agents, and calcium channel blockers.

Clinical Conference Activities

- Regardless of the medical diagnosis of the assigned client, ask students to share their assessment findings. Have conference group discuss the significance of these findings.
- Ask students to discuss how monitoring enzyme levels can help the nurse to make nursing decisions regarding the care of a client with an MI.
- Ask students to discuss their experiences in the cardiac rehabilitation unit. (See Clinical Site Activities.) Ask each student to identify a nursing diagnosis and two related nursing interventions appropriate for a client observed in the unit.
- Ask a dietitian to talk to students about dietary management of atherosclerosis. Assign students to develop a dietary plan directed toward limiting atherosclerosis.

- Ask students to describe a diagnostic study that facilitated the diagnosis of their assigned client.
- Invite a dietitian to discuss low-sodium diets. Ask the dietitian to apply dietary principles to the clients assigned to the students.
- Assign groups of students to visit the American Heart Association and have them share their findings in clinical conference.
- Assign each student to select a drug on the crash cart. Ask the student to share in conference the reason for administration, pharmacologic actions, major side effects, and nursing implications.
- Demonstrate a defibrillator to the conference group. Discuss paddle placement and nursing responsibilities during a cardiac arrest.
- Assign each student to bring a journal article on ethical issues related to cardiac disorders; e.g., use of pacemakers, institution of CPR and do not resuscitate (DNR) orders.
- Discuss with students home healthcare issues associated with MI rehabilitation.

CHAPTER

46

Nursing Care of Clients with Disorders of Cardiac Rhythm

Objectives

46.1 Define the terms related to disorders of cardiac rhythm.

46.2 Trace the cardiac conduction system.

46.3 Identify the components of the electrocardiogram (ECG) pattern.

46.4 Interpret selected rhythm strips.

46.5 Discuss the medical management of selected dysrhythmias.

46.6 Describe the management of life-threatening dysrhythmias.

46.7 Discuss the surgical management of dysrhythmias.

46.8 Discuss the major nursing interventions related to disorders of the cardiac rhythm.

Facilitating Student Learning

CLASSROOM

Review Activity

- Ask students to review Chapter 43.

Class Assignments

- Assign students to complete Chapter 46 in the Study Guide prior to class.
- Ask the students to explain why the nurse's observations and assessments are important in the care of a client with cardiac dysrhythmias.
- Ask students to make copies of the dysrhythmia note-taking outline in the Study Guide to use in class.

Lecture/Discussion

- Review the cardiac conduction system.
- Explain the three major mechanisms of dysrhythmias: automaticity, conduction, and problems with reentry impulses.
- Explain the classification of dysrhythmias according to where they arise in the conduction system: SA node, atria, AV node, and ventricles.
- Explain what is meant by *intrinsic rates of conduction*.
- Review the normal ECG pattern and correlate each phase with the cardiac cycle.
- Demonstrate how to use the basic step to interpret rhythm strips.
- Allow time for students to practice labeling the parts of the ECG waveform and measuring them.
- Refer students to Table 46–1 and Box 46–1. Recommend that the students make a copy of these to use as references.
- Organize the lecture content according to where the dysrhythmias originate in the heart. Use the dysrhythmia note-taking outline as a guide.
- Depending on the level of the students and unit objectives, focus on etiology, identification, clinical manifestations, and treatment of cardiac dysrhythmias.
- Present a case study of a client with a cardiac dysrhythmia. Ask students to develop nursing diagnoses, collaborative problems, expected outcomes, and nursing interventions based on the assessment data.
- Present a case study of a client with a permanent pacemaker. Ask students to develop nursing diagnoses, collaborative problems, goals, expected outcomes, and nursing interventions based on the assessed data.
- Present a case study of a client with a permanent pacemaker. Refer students to Appendix D7, Coordinated CareMap for a Pacemaker. Use this CareMap as a guide to illustrate concept of coordinated care. Give assessment data that correlates with the CareMap and the case study. Focus on rationales for interventions and evaluation of the goals and outcome criteria. Ask the students to describe how they will know the goals are being met. (You may have to clarify that outcome criteria/expected outcomes are the AEB listed under the goals. You may have to review the evaluation process.)
- Discuss treatment of life-threatening dysrhythmias.

Transparencies

- Figure 43–9—The Cardiac Conduction System
- Normal ECG Pattern (Study Guide)
- 82(M)—Normal Sinus Rhythm
- 83(M)—Disturbances in Atrial Impulse Generation
- 84(M)—Premature Junctional Contraction
- 85(M)—Disturbances in Junctional Conduction

- 86(M)—Disorder Arising in the Ventricles
- 87(M)—Transvenous Catheter Placement
- Table 46–1—Risk Factors and Level of Prevention
- Box 46–1—Electrocardiographic Interpretation of Dysrhythmias

Group Activity

- Divide the students in small groups. Provide each group with ECG tracings. Ask the students to use Box 46–1 and Table 46–1 as guides to interpret the rhythms.

CLINICAL

Skills Laboratory

- Create a mock code situation where students quickly identify life-threatening dysrhythmias and simulate CPR.

Clinical Site Activities

- Assign students to care for clients with disorders of cardiac rhythm.
- In postconference, give students a brief case study and mystery rhythm strip to identify. Discuss possible etiology, clinical manifestations, and treatment.
- Assign students to submit an interpreted rhythm strip each week.
- Make arrangements for students to obtain a rhythm strip from a telemetry unit or coronary care unit if the students' clients are not being monitored.
- Create a *Jeopardy*-type game to use in class or postconference. Develop categories that relate to the students' level and objectives of the course. Be creative! Suggestions:

  —Pharmacy

  —Patient data

  —Point of origin

  —Prognosis

  —Picture strips

CHAPTER

47

Nursing Care of Clients with Disorders of Cardiac Structure

Objectives

47.1 Describe the predisposing factors, pathophysiology, etiology, clinical manifestations, and complications for the disorders that are the result of an inflammatory response.

47.2 Describe the predisposing factors, pathophysiology, etiology, clinical manifestations, and complications for selected structural abnormalities of the heart.

47.3 Describe the pathophysiologic changes that occur with cardiac tamponade.

47.4 Describe medical management and nursing care of clients with cardiac conditions.

47.5 Describe the surgical management and nursing care for selected cardiac disorders.

47.6 Identify postoperative collaborative problems that may occur with cardiac surgery.

Facilitating Student Learning

CLASSROOM

Review Activities

- Assign students to review Chapter 45 for techniques used to monitor central venous pressure, arterial pressure, and pulmonary artery pressure. Encourage the students to go to the Psychomotor Skills Laboratory to look at the monitoring equipment used with these procedures.
- Assign students to review Chapter 21 for content on perioperative nursing care.

Class Assignments

- Assign students to complete Chapter 47 of the Study Guide before class.
- Use role playing to demonstrate the teaching of techniques needed to administer intravenous antibiotics at home.
- Assign students to develop a 24-hour dietary plan for an individual with rheumatic fever.
- Assign selected students to discuss medical therapy for an individual with infective endocarditis. Ask the class to discuss rationales for the medical therapy and related nursing responsibilities.
- Present a case study of an individual with infective endocarditis. Ask the students to identify goals, nursing diagnoses, and nursing interventions based on assessed data.
- Assign students to listen to simulated heart sounds: normal sounds, pericardial friction rubs, and murmurs.
- Supply students with three case studies of individuals with structural heart disorders. Ask the students to identify the subjective and objective manifestations of each disorder.
- Ask students to explain how the following conditions might precipitate cardiomyopathy:
  1. Last trimester of pregnancy
  2. Polycythemia vera
  3. Amyloidosis
  4. Collagen disease
  5. Obesity
  6. Viral infections
- Supply students with a case study of an individual with congestive cardiomyopathy. Ask the students to identify appropriate nursing diagnoses and nursing goals.
- Present a case study of an individual in the preextubation period following cardiac surgery. Assign students to identify appropriate nursing diagnoses, goals, and nursing interventions based on assessed data.
- Use role playing to demonstrate discharge teaching of an individual following cardiac surgery. Ask students to include dietary restrictions, activity needs, incision care, pulse monitoring, and follow-up care with the physician.
- Ask students to discuss how monitoring each of the following provides information needed to plan appropriate nursing interventions for the person in the postoperative phase of cardiac surgery:
  1. Apical-radial pulse
  2. Body temperature
  3. Chest drainage
  4. Intake and output
  5. Urine color
  6. Level of consciousness
  7. Tolerance for activity
  8. Psychologic status

- Ask students to bring a newspaper or nonprofessional magazine article on the subject of heart surgery. Discuss these articles in class focusing on the quality of information being distributed to the public.

Lecture/Discussion

- This chapter contains many important concepts. Allow sufficient time for coverage of the material and assimilation of the content.
- Discuss the pathology of the inflammatory process. Stress the tissue/organ changes that occur as a result of inflammation.
- Focus presentation on pathophysiology of rheumatic fever, infective endocarditis, myocarditis, and pericarditis.
- Discuss the major drug groups used to treat inflammatory cardiovascular (CV) diseases. Select one drug that typifies each group and discuss it in depth.
- Focus the discussion on nursing measures specific for an individual with an inflammatory CV disease. Ask students to supply the rationales for these measures.
- Discuss the pathophysiologic changes that occur with a cardiac tamponade.
- Focus the lecture on the pathophysiology of CV structural disorders. Emphasize the common pathologic changes that exist among the numerous conditions. For example, in all cardiomyopathies the cardiac function is impaired because the disease process affects cardiac muscle fibers. Knowledge of pathophysiology will help students to deduce subjective and objective manifestations.
- Discuss nursing measures specific for individuals with cardiomyopathy or valvular heart disease. Ask students to supply the rationales for these measures.
- Discuss briefly the three major types of open-heart surgery discussed in this chapter.
- Discuss briefly the purpose of hypothermia and extracorporeal circulation.
- Focus the lecture on assessment and care of the individual following open-heart surgery.
- Use Appendix D6, Coordinated CareMap for open-heart and valve surgery to emphasize the collaborative type of care plans and the nurse's role in implementing and evaluating the care plan.

Transparencies

- 88(T)—Manifestations of Subacute Bacterial Endocarditis (Figure 43–3)
- 89(T)—Types of Cardiomyopathy (Figure 43–5)
- Mitral Valve Prolapse (Figure 47–6)
- 91(T)—Mitral Stenosis
- 92(T)—Mitral Insufficiency
- 93(T)—Aortic Stenosis
- 94(T)—Aortic Insufficiency

Group Activities

- Divide the class into small groups. Provide each group with a case study of an individual with infective endocarditis. Assign the groups to develop a learning/teaching plan that includes one or more of the following: purpose of long-term antibiotic administration, procedure for administering antibiotics, activity restriction, self-assessment for manifestations of endocarditis, oral hygiene needs, and need for prophylactic antibiotics. After the group work, ask the groups to present their plans to the class and to explain the rationales for the measures included on the plans.
- Divide the students into small groups. Supply each group with a case study of a client with a valvular heart disease. Assign the students to develop a plan of care for this individual. Ask them to share their plans and the rationales for their decisions with the entire class.

- Divide the class into five groups and provide each group one of the following items of assessment data:
  —Appears tense, quiet, and relies on spouse for support
  —WBC 18,000/mm; redness and pain at incision site
  —Perspiring, rapid pulse, productive cough, temperature at 38° C
  —Incisional pain, hesitancy to cough and deep breathe
  —Restless, cannot remember day or date, questions the meaning of all conversation occurring in the room
- Ask the groups to discuss the significance of the finding in the postextubation period. Assign the students to discuss the medical and nursing interventions appropriate in each situation.

Guest Speakers

- Invite a dietitian to class to discuss a diet appropriate for an individual with rheumatic fever, such as a high-protein, high-carbohydrate diet.
- Invite a nurse clinical specialist to discuss the effects of a CV structural disorder on the client's growth and development. Ask the speaker to stress how the nurse can promote normal growth and development.
- Invite a CV clinical specialist to class to discuss the pre- and postoperative nursing care associated with cardiac surgery.
- Invite a CV clinical specialist to class to discuss using a clinical pathway/CareMap with clients undergoing cardiac surgery.

CLINICAL

Skills Laboratory

- Demonstrate how to check for a paradoxical pulse.
- Demonstrate procedure for performing a pericardiocentesis.
- Review monitoring and maintenance of chest tubes.
- Demonstrate/return demonstrate cardiovascular assessment.

Clinical Site Activities

- Assign students to assess a client who has an inflammatory heart disease. (If this is not possible, check CV histories to determine individuals with postinflammatory heart disorders and assign them to students.)
- Assign students to assess for a paradoxical pulse on their assigned clients.
- Ask students to check records of an assigned client for leukocyte count and sedimentation rate.
- Ask students to develop a care plan based on assessed data. Have the students include in the care plan goals, nursing diagnoses, expected outcomes, and nursing interventions.
- Ask students to give rationales for specific nursing interventions included in the care plan.
- Assign students to develop drug cards that include pharmacologic action, expected physiologic response, side effects, usual dosage, route of administration, and nursing implications for selected medications used in the medical management of cardiac disorders.

- Assign students to develop a discharge plan that considers diet, drugs, exercise, and activities.
- Assign students to assess a client with a structural heart disorder or valvular heart disease. (Since many of these medical diagnoses are associated with the young, these experiences should be assigned during a nursing of children clinical rotation if possible.)
- Assign students to assess a client with cardiomyopathy or a condition that can precipitate cardiomyopathy.
- Assign students to observe in an adult or pediatric CV clinic.
- If possible, assign students to assess a client scheduled for cardiac surgery. Ask students to identify appropriate nursing diagnoses and nursing interventions for this client.
- Assign students to assess a client following cardiac surgery. (It would be ideal if students could follow the same individual through the preoperative, intraoperative, and postoperative periods.)
- Assign students to observe open-heart surgery.
- Assign students to observe in the recovery room and/or ICU the care of the client following cardiac surgery.
- Assign students to assess a client who has had previous heart surgery. Ask the students to focus assessment on the individual's recall of and response to the surgery.

Clinical Conference Activities

- Ask students to share their assessment findings. Ask the conference group to discuss the significance of the findings.
- Ask students to identify the diagnostic procedures used to confirm the CV disease in their assigned client.
- Invite a cardiac clinical specialist to discuss cardiac changes associated with inflammatory CV disorders: arrhythmias, heart gallops, and murmurs.
- Ask students to discuss their experiences in the CV clinic (see Clinical Site Activities). Ask each student to identify one nursing diagnosis and two related nursing interventions appropriate for an individual observed in the clinic.
- Invite a therapist to conference to discuss chest physiotherapy. Ask the therapist to discuss techniques that can be used on the client following surgery involving the chest cavity.
- Ask students to discuss their operating room, recovery room, and/or ICU observation experiences (see Clinical Site Activities).
- Play an audio- or videotape of various heart sounds and have the students name the sound and discuss the etiology and treatment.

CHAPTER

48

Structure and Function of the Peripheral Vascular System

Objectives

48.1 Discuss the major terms related to the peripheral vascular system.

48.2 Identify the major structures of the peripheral vascular system.

48.3 Discuss the functions of the peripheral vascular system.

48.4 Explain the mechanisms that maintain arterial blood pressure.

48.5 Discuss blood flow through the tissues.

48.6 Discuss the effect of aging on the peripheral vascular system.

Facilitating Student Learning

CLASSROOM

Class Assignment

- Assign students to complete Chapter 48 in the Study Guide before class.

Lecture/Discussion

- Review the structure and function of the peripheral vascular system. Use Transparencies 75(T), 76(T), 80(T), and 95(T).
- Review the factors that regulate the peripheral vascular system: nervous system, hormonal system, chemical substances, and local regulatory mechanisms.
- Discuss physiologic effect of the sympathetic nervous system and renin-angiotensin-aldosterone system on vasomotor activity. Use Transparency 95(T) to clarify content.
- Review the structure and function of the lymphatic system. Use Figure 48–5 to clarify content.

Transparencies

- 75(T)—Major Arteries
- 76(T)—Major Veins
- 80(T)—Cross-Section of Artery and Vein
- 95(T)—Role of Renin-Angiotensin-Aldosterone System in Regulation of Blood Pressure
- 99(M)—Venous Return from the Legs
- Figure 48–2—Cross-Sections of an Artery and Vein
- Figure 48–4—One-Way Venous Valves
- Figure 48–5—Superficial Lymphatic System

CHAPTER

49

Assessment of Clients with Peripheral Vascular Disorders

OBJECTIVES

49.1 Describe important assessment data to obtain during the peripheral vascular nursing history.

49.2 Discuss signs and symptoms associated with peripheral vascular disorders.

49.3 Perform basic physical assessment of the peripheral vascular system.

49.4 Describe pathophysiologic bases for selected assessment data.

49.5 Describe pre- and postprocedure nursing care of selected noninvasive and invasive diagnostic techniques.

Facilitating Student Learning

CLASSROOM

Class Assignments

- Assign students to complete Chapter 49 in the Study Guide before class.
- Assign students to review Chapter 48 on the structure and function of the peripheral vascular system.

Lecture/Discussion

- Review the structure and function of the peripheral vascular system as needed.
- Focus a lecture on pertinent aspects of a peripheral vascular history. Use the framework developed by your school to make it easier for students to understand.
- Emphasize the focused physical examination. Use the mnemonic "8 Ps" of the peripheral vascular assessment.
- Compare and contrast the clinical manifestations of arterial and venous disorders. Use Table 49-1.
- Explain the concept and etiology of edema. Use Figure 49-1 to explain the edema assessment.
- Discuss assessing peripheral pulses. Use Figure 49 or the example in the Study Guide to clarify content.
- Demonstrate the Homan's sign and Allen's test. Discuss possible implications of the tests.
- Discuss the diagnostic tests related to the peripheral vascular system. Emphasize the concept of invasive versus noninvasive tests and the nursing responsibilities.

Group Activities

- Provide students with a list of clinical manifestations of peripheral vascular disorders. Have the students categorize them under arterial or venous.
- Divide the students into small groups. Assign each group a diagnostic test, and have the students develop a 5-minute teaching plan to present to the class.

CLINICAL

Skills Laboratory

- Demonstrate an assessment of the peripheral vascular system and include a health history and a physical exam.
- Discuss the use of a scale to determine the extent of edema and pallor.
- Demonstrate assessment of peripheral pulses. Discuss the scale used to grade peripheral pulses.
- Demonstrate the Homan's sign and Allen's test.
- Demonstrate the use of Doppler ultrasound flow meter.
- Demonstrate funduscopic examination. Emphasize retinopathy associated with hypertension. Provide colored photographs that exemplify the changes in the retina.
- Demonstrate wrapping of above- and below-knee stumps and above-elbow stumps.

Clinical Site Activities

- Assign students to obtain a peripheral vascular nursing history and perform a physical assessment on an assigned client.
- If possible, assign students to assess clients with an arterial disorder and a venous disorder. Have the students compare and contrast their findings.
- Arrange for students to observe exercise tests for intermittent claudication and or angiography for peripheral arterial disease.
- Assign students to prepare a discharge plan for a client with peripheral arterial occlusive disease and chronic venous disease. Ask students to consider wound and ulcer care, early identification of complications, ambulation, and diet.

Clinical Conference Activities

- Ask students to share assessment findings on their clients.
- Ask students to share the problems identified for their clients. Guide the students in a discussion of common problems, nursing diagnoses, and nursing responsibilities.
- Discuss clinical pathways or Care Maps used by the clinical facility. Emphasize the problems, nursing diagnoses, and nursing responsibilities common to both comprehensive and collaborative plans of care.
- Have students evaluate a case study of a client's progress toward meeting the goals and expected outcomes. Include abnormal laboratory and diagnostic test data for students to analyze.
- Ask students to discuss what should be included in teaching/learning guidelines for clients with peripheral vascular disease.

CHAPTER

50

Nursing Care of Clients with Peripheral Vascular Disorders

Objectives

50.1 Identify and describe the major classifications of hypertension.

50.2 Identify primary and secondary prevention measures for primary hypertension.

50.3 Discuss incidence, risk factors, etiology, clinical manifestations, and pathophysiology of primary hypertension.

50.4 Describe possible complications of hypertension.

50.5 Describe nonpharmacologic medical management of primary hypertension.

50.6 Describe the pharmacologic action, expected response, side effects, and nursing considerations of drugs used to treat hypertension: diuretics, sympatholytic agents, vasodilators, angiotensin-converting enzyme inhibitors, and calcium channel blockers.

50.7 Differentiate between acute and chronic arterial disorders and acute and chronic venous disorders.

50.8 Summarize the etiology, risk factors, pathophysiology, complications, and medical and surgical treatment of peripheral vascular disorders.

50.9 Discuss the nursing management of the client with peripheral vascular disorders.

50.10 Discuss the nursing management of the surgical client undergoing percutaneous transluminal angioplasty, arterial bypass, amputation, and abdominal aortic aneurysm surgery.

Facilitating Student Learning

CLASSROOM

Review Activities

- Assign students to review Chapter 48 on the structures and functions of the peripheral vascular system and the lymphatic system.
- Assign students to review Chapter 49 on assessment of clients with peripheral vascular disorders.

Class Assignments

- Assign students to complete Chapter 50 in the Study Guide before class.
- Assign selected students to discuss in class one of the following factors that regulates the peripheral vascular system: nervous system, hormonal system and chemical substances, and local regulatory mechanisms.
- Assign students to monitor the blood pressure of another individual (spouse, classmate, family member, etc.). The blood pressure should be taken at various times during a 24-hour period and following activities such as smoking, drinking, consuming beverages that contain caffeine, exercising, and relaxing. Ask students to record their findings on a graph and be prepared to discuss any significant findings.
- Assign students to check labels of food for sodium content. Ask them to list those items with high sodium content.

Lecture/Discussion

Hypertension

- Have the students review the blood pressure assignment (see Class Assignments) and write down what they believe caused the variations in the blood pressure readings (time limit: two minutes).
- List the main factors that regulate blood pressure on an overhead or blackboard. Ask for volunteers to discuss the assignment findings and what they believe caused the variations. Categorize their answers under the main factors.
- Review the structure and function of the peripheral vascular system. Use Transparencies 75(T), 76(T), and 80(T).
- Present a case study on hypertension that includes all phases of diagnosis, treatment, and complications of hypertension.
- Ask students to differentiate between primary and secondary hypertension. Use Box 50–1, Causes of Secondary Hypertension.
- Review the pathophysiology and clinical manifestations of primary hypertension.
- Discuss the medical treatment for hypertension and explain the step program.
- Guide the students in a discussion of how lifestyle changes can reduce blood pressure.
- Discuss the major drug groups used to treat hypertension. Select one drug that typifies each group and discuss this drug in depth.
- Discuss hypertensive crisis and the medications used in the treatment of the disorder.

Peripheral Vascular Disorders

- Two-minute paper: ask the students to write down their understanding of the terms *acute* and *chronic*.
- Ask the students to divide a piece of paper into four sections. Label the top sections "acute arterial disorders" and "acute venous disorders." Label the bottom two sections "chronic arterial disorders" and "chronic venous disorders." Allow one minute for each section, then ask the students to write down what they know about each section.
- Lead the students in a discussion of the assignment. Review the structure and function of the peripheral vascular system as needed.
- Present a case study of selected acute and chronic arterial disorders.
- Discuss the pathophysiology of selected arterial or venous disorders. Have the students discuss the medical and nursing management of these disorders.

- Discuss the risk factors for each disorder.
- Discuss the clinical manifestations for each disorder.
- Discuss the medical and/or surgical treatment for these disorders.
- Discuss acute arterial and venous thrombus formation. Compare and contrast each type of disorder. Ask the students to discuss the treatment of the disorders.
- Emphasize the nursing responsibilities.
- Focus on the types of amputation procedures, levels of amputation, and the immediate postoperative prosthesis fitting. Use Transparency 97(T) to clarify the information.
- Obtain a prosthesis to show the students.

Transparencies

- 75(T)—Major Arteries
- 76 (T)—Major Veins
- 80 (T)—Cross-Section of Artery and Vein
- 95(T)—Role of Renin-Angiotensin-Aldosterone System in Regulation of Blood Pressure.
- 96(T)—Classifications of Aneurysms
- 97 (M)—Common Sites of Amputations
- 98(T)—Femoral Artery Bypass Grafts
- 99 (M)—Venous Return from the Legs
- 100 (M)—Types of Lymphedema
- Box 50–1—Causes of Secondary Hypertension
- Box 50–2—Stepped Care Approach to Management of Hypertension

Group Activities

- Divide the class into small groups. Provide each group with a typical diet for a nursing student. Ask the students to figure the sodium content and compare it with the recommended daily amount of sodium.
- If time permits, have each student complete an individual diet analysis for sodium content.
- Divide the class into small groups and provide each group with a case study of a client with peripheral arterial occlusive disease, deep vein thrombosis (DVT), and lymphatic disorder. Ask the students to identify the clinical manifestations, diagnostic tests, and complications of each disorder and to develop a comprehensive plan of care.
- Provide a clinical pathway/CareMap for arterial bypass surgery or amputation. Provide assessment data and lab data for selected postoperative days. Have the students evaluate the client's progress toward meeting the goals and expected outcomes.

Guest Speakers

- Invite appropriate healthcare workers to discuss stress management methods (e.g., biofeedback and relaxation techniques) that may be helpful for the hypertensive client.
- Invite a dietitian to talk about low-sodium, low-fat, low-cholesterol, and calorie-restricted diets. Ask the dietitian to discuss techniques for adapting the diet to meet the client's personal, religious, and cultural preferences.
- Invite prosthetists to class to discuss prosthetic fitting and training.
- Invite a therapist from the rehabilitation unit to class to discuss postamputation rehabilitation.
- Invite a head nurse or someone from one of the nursing units to discuss using clinical pathways/coordinated CareMaps.

CLINICAL

Skills Laboratory

- Demonstrate a peripheral vascular assessment.
- Demonstrate the use of a Doppler.

Clinical Site Activities

- Assign students to participate in a community hypertension screening program.
- Assign students to care for a client with primary hypertension. (This may not be the client's primary diagnosis.) Have the students develop a comprehensive plan of care for this client, including a teaching plan.

- If hypertension is not the primary medical diagnosis, ask the students to discuss how hypertension affects or is affected by the primary diagnosis.
- Assign students to care for a client with an arterial, venous, or lymphatic disorder.
- Have the students complete a health history and physical assessment. Ask students to develop a comprehensive care plan based on assessed data. Include rationales for the nursing diagnosis and nursing interventions.
- Have the students compare and contrast their client's clinical manifestations, diagnostic tests, complications, and medical/surgical treatment with a classical textbook picture of the medical diagnosis.
- If a clinical pathway is available, have the students evaluate the client's progress toward meeting the expected outcomes.
- Depending on the focus of the clinical experience and the level of the student, the clinical pathway may be used instead of a comprehensive care plan.

Clinical Conference Activities

- Assign students to do a walking grand rounds of their clients. The level and complexity of the assignment can vary: compare and contrast to classical textbook picture, clinical manifestations, medications, etc.
- Ask students to share assessment findings on their clients. Ask the group to discuss the significance of these findings.
- Assign students to do a postconference teaching project on an aspect of a peripheral vascular disorder. Assign these topics at the beginning of the clinical rotation.
- Have students "present a client" in postconference. Develop guidelines based on the course and level objectives.
- Assign the students a short five-minute reflective paper on an aspect of the clinical experience.
- At the beginning of each clinical conference activity, explain the purpose and expectations. At the end of each clinical conference, take a few minutes to debrief and tie everything together.

CHAPTER

51

Structure and Function of the Hematologic System

Objectives

51.1 Discuss normal structure and function of blood and the components of blood.

51.2 Explain the hematopoietic process.

51.3 Discuss blood groups and blood typing.

51.4 Explain the relationship among the ABO, Rh, and HLA systems and blood compatibility.

51.5 Discuss the three phases of homeostasis.

51.6 Discuss the effects of aging on the hematologic system.

Facilitating Student Learning

CLASSROOM

Review Activity

- Assign students to review notes and/or anatomy-physiology textbook for information on blood group systems.

Class Assignments

- Assign students to complete Chapter 51 in the Study Guide before class.
- Assign selected students to discuss in class one of the functions of blood described in this chapter.
- Assign a student to visit the local American Red Cross. Have the student determine donor selection procedure, number of pints of blood donated during the past year, changes in procedures that have occurred since the outbreak of AIDS, peak time of year for blood donations, etc.
- Ask students to develop a meal plan that would increase the intake of iron and folic acid.

Lecture/Discussion

- Most of this material was probably covered in an anatomy-physiology course. Therefore, it should be presented in a review or discussion format.
- Ask the students to discuss the characteristics of blood.
- Review hematopoiesis and erythropoiesis.
- Review the ABO, Rh, and HLA systems. Stress the antigen-antibody reactions associated with each system.
- Review hemostasis; use Transparencies 101(T) and 102(T) to clarify this process.

Transparencies

- 101(T)—Formed Elements in the Blood
- 102(T)—Development of the Formed Elements
- Figure 51-2—Regulation of Erythrocyte Production
- Figure 51-3—Development of Lymphocytes
- Figure 51-4—Cell-Mediated Immunity
- Figure 51-5—Antibody-Mediated Immunity
- Figure 51-6—Mechanism of Normal Homeostasis
- Figure 51-7—The Coagulation Process
- Figure 51-8—Fibrin Enmeshing a Red Blood Cell

CHAPTER

52

Assessment of Clients with Hematologic Disorders

OBJECTIVES

52.1 Identify normal values for adult complete blood count (CBC) and differential count.

52.2 List the four basic pathophysiologic disturbances that characterize hematologic disorders.

52.3 Describe aspects to include in the nursing history and physical assessment of clients with hematologic disorders.

52.4 Describe the diagnostic studies and associated nursing interventions used to confirm or differentiate hematologic disorders.

Facilitating Student Learning

CLASSROOM

Review Activity

- Assign students to review function and structure of the hematopoietic system in Chapter 51.

Class Assignments

- Assign students to complete Chapter 52 in the Study Guide before class.
- Assign selected students to discuss in class one of the functions of blood described in this chapter.

Lecture/Discussion

- Review basic terminology related to hematologic disorders.
- Review function of each blood element.
- Focus a lecture on analyzing a CBC, red blood cell indices, and a white blood cell count (WBC) with differential. Distribute copies of lab work for students to analyze using a laboratory manual.
- Use the data assessment framework for your school to guide students in the pertinent information to gather.
- Divide students into small groups. Give each group a different case study with a client undergoing a bone marrow aspiration. Guide the students in a discussion of the indications for a bone marrow aspiration and the nursing care involved.

CLINICAL

Skills Laboratory

- Demonstrate and practice phlebotomy. If possible, run a CBC on each student.
- Demonstrate taking a health history and physical assessment of a client with a hematologic disorder.
- Ask students to type their own blood. This gives the students the opportunity to observe agglutination.
- Demonstrate and have students practice assessment of the hematologic system.

Clinical Site Activities

- Have students find a complete blood count on a client's chart. Have them practice reading it and differentiating normal from abnormal findings.
- Assign students to visit the hospital's blood bank. Ask the technician in charge of the blood bank to describe the procedures used for blood storage and blood typing and cross-matching.
- Assign students to clients who are scheduled for diagnostic studies related to the hematologic system. Have students prepare the client for the test and perform postprocedure care.
- Ask students to complete an assessment of the hematologic system on an assigned client.

Clinical Conference Activities

- Assign students to review institutional policies for ordering, handling, and administering blood and blood products. Discuss these policies and their impact on nursing care.
- Ask students to share their assessment findings. Have the group develop appropriate nursing diagnoses, expected outcomes, and interventions for one client.

CHAPTER

53

Nursing Care of Clients with Hematologic Disorders

Objectives

53.1 Describe the two basic pathophysiologic alterations that underlie all red blood cell disorders.

53.2 Describe etiology, pathophysiology, clinical manifestations, diagnostic studies, and complications of selected erythrocyte disorders.

53.3 Describe the medical and surgical management of clients with various hematologic disorders.

53.4 Describe nursing care of clients with various hematologic disorders.

53.5 Provide rationales for nursing care of the client requiring a blood transfusion.

53.6 Evaluate effectiveness of care based on expected outcomes.

Facilitating Student Learning

CLASSROOM

Review Activities

- Assign students to review content on normal erythrocyte structure, function, and life span in an anatomy-physiology textbook.
- Assign students to review the hemostatic mechanism and the structure and function of leukocytes and plasma cells.
- Ask students to review Chapter 52 on diagnostic studies associated with hematologic disorders.
- Assign students to review an anatomy and physiology textbook on blood group systems.

Class Assignments

- Assign students to complete Chapter 53 in the Study Guide before class.
- Supply students with a case study of a client with anemia. Ask students to identify the subjective and objective manifestations and the type of anemia.
- Provide students with the manifestations listed below; ask them to provide the pathophysiologic bases for each.

  —Palpitations

  —Sensitivity to cold

  —Dizziness

  —Fatigue

  —Angina pectoris

  —Congestive heart failure
- Ask students to develop a discharge plan for an individual with an erythrocyte disorder that considers the following: drugs, diet, safety measures, hygiene, and comfort measures.
- Provide the students with a list of clinical manifestations of acute leukemia, chronic myelogenous leukemia, or chronic lymphocytic leukemia. Ask students to provide the pathophysiologic bases for these manifestations.
- Ask students to plan one day's food intake for an individual with stomatitis.
- Supply students with a case study of a client experiencing a hemolytic reaction. Have students identify the subjective and objective manifestations of the reaction.
- Have students select a hematologic disorder that they want to study in more depth. Assign students to find two journal articles that address the disorder (one of the articles should be a nursing research study). Ask the students to share findings with the class.

Lecture/Discussion

- Start this portion of study by asking the students to describe normal erythrocyte structure, function, and life span. Ask them to provide the normal values for red blood cell count, hemoglobin, hematocrit, and reticulocyte count.
- Review the diagnostic tests used to determine abnormal erythrocyte structure, function, and life span.
- Since there are numerous types of anemia, you need to determine the focus of the class session. This section in the textbook is divided into acquired, traumatic, and congenital disorders. In class session, present one disorder from each category in depth.
- Before presenting the three types of anemia in depth, you should begin by discussing the common pathologic changes that exist among the various anemias. Emphasize the common manifestations that exist among the anemias. Also include the medical management of anemias, including oxygen therapy, blood transfusions, drug therapy, and diet therapy.

- Obtain slides that depict the structural changes in erythrocytes that occur in selected disorders.
- Discuss the major drug groups used to treat erythrocyte disorders. Select one drug that typifies each group and discuss this drug in depth.
- Discuss disorders that cause overproduction of red blood cells. Emphasize the pathology produced by excessive circulating red blood cells.
- Start this portion of study by asking the students to describe normal leukocyte structure, function, and life span. Ask them to provide you with the normal values for white blood cell count and differential count.
- Since the signs and symptoms of all types of leukemia are similar, discuss common clinical manifestations and the associated pathogenesis. Briefly mention the specific diagnostic studies used to differentiate the types of leukemia. Focus on the nurse's role in the medical/surgical management of leukemia.
- Use case study approach to study agranulocytosis and multiple myeloma (see Group Activities).
- Differentiate between Hodgkin's disease and non-Hodgkin's lymphoma. The case study approach to study Hodgkin's disease can be used; concentrate a class session on non-Hodgkin's lymphoma and infectious mononucleosis. Include the staging classification of Hodgkin's disease.
- Review the hemostatic mechanism.
- As with the erythrocyte and leukocyte disorders, concentrate on the commonalties among the disorders of platelets and clotting factors. Since many conditions can precipitate disseminated intravascular coagulation (DIC), more time should be spent discussing this condition.
- Sickle-cell anemia and hemophilias are probably discussed in material on nursing of children. Stress the impact of these conditions on the adult.

Transparencies

- 103(T)—Hodgkin's Disease

Guest Speaker

- Invite an oncology nurse to class to discuss the chemotherapeutic agents used in the treatment of leukemias and lymphomas. Ask the nurse to discuss specific nursing interventions related to the drug therapy.

Group Activities

- Divide the class into small groups. Ask students to discuss how the following factors might cause anemia.

  —Vitamin B_{12} deficiency

  —Intrinsic factor deficiency

  —Radiation therapy

  —Severed blood vessels due to trauma

  —Iron deficiency

  —Lead poisoning

- Divide the class into small groups. Ask students to discuss how the following diagnostic tests confirm erythrocyte disorders.

  —Erythrocyte indices

  —Urobilinogen test

  —Schilling's test

  —Gastric secretion analysis

  —Serum folate level

  —Bone marrow examination

- Divide the class into six groups. Provide each group with a case study on one of the following: chronic myelogenous leukemia, agranulocytosis, multiple myeloma, Hodgkin's disease, idiopathic thrombocytopenia purpura, and hemophilia A. Ask students to identify the clinical manifestations found in the case study. Have them discuss etiologies, pathophysiology, diagnostic tests, and clinical interventions for each disorder.

- Divide the class into small groups. Ask each group to develop a learning/teaching guide for one of the following:
  —Potential for infection due to low granulocyte count
  —Potential for bleeding due to thrombocytopenia
  —Potential for injury due to osteoporosis
- Ask students to consider how these guidelines would be altered for a client in each of the developmental stages.

CLINICAL

Skills Laboratory

- Role play teaching a client to self-administer vitamin B_{12} injections.
- Demonstrate bone marrow aspiration procedure.
- Demonstrate Z-track or air-lock injection technique.
- Discuss blood transfusions. Discuss informed consent, pretransfusion testing, and blood bank regulations. Demonstrate blood infusion equipment and devices. Discuss monitoring the client and nursing management of transfusion reactions.

Clinical Site Activities

- Assign students to assess an individual with a major hematologic disorder. Based on their assessed data, have the students develop a comprehensive plan of care.
- Ask students to provide the rationale for specific nursing interventions included on the care plan.
- Assign students to develop drug cards that include pharmacologic action, expected physiologic response, side effects, usual dosage, route of administration, and nursing implications for selected chemotherapeutic agents.
- Arrange for students to observe chemotherapy administration.
- Assign students to determine if community resources related to erythrocyte disorders exist; for instance, sickle cell anemia screening.
- Assign students to visit the hospital's blood bank. Ask the technician in charge of the blood bank to describe the procedures used for blood storage and blood typing and cross-matching.

Clinical Conference Activities

- Ask students to share their assessment findings; have the conference group discuss the significance of these findings.
- Ask students to identify the diagnostic studies that confirmed the existence of a hematologic disorder in their client.
- Invite the dietitian to conference; ask the individual to give examples of meals with higher-than-normal amounts of protein, iron, vitamins, and minerals.
- Ask the dietitian to discuss methods of promoting proper nutrition for a client experiencing side effects from chemotherapy or radiation therapy.
- Discuss the relationship among erythrocyte disorders, activities, and metabolic needs. Ask the students to discuss how nurses can intervene to reduce oxygen requirements of the client with an erythrocyte disorder.
- Ask students to discuss their observational experience (see Clinical Site Activities). Ask students to identify one nursing diagnosis and two nursing interventions specific to one of the clients receiving chemotherapy.

- Ask students to provide the purpose, normal values, and finding interpretation for the following laboratory studies used to diagnose hemorrhagic disorders:

  —Bleeding time

  —Prothrombin time

  —Platelet count

  —Partial thromboplastin time

  —Clotting time

  —Rumple-Leeds test

- Assign students to review institutional policies for ordering, handling, and administering blood and blood products. Discuss these policies and their impact on nursing care.

CHAPTER

54

Structure and Function of the Urinary System

OBJECTIVES

54.1 Describe the structure and function of the normal urinary tract.

54.2 Identify the two main functions of the urinary system.

54.3 Describe the process of urine formation.

54.4 Describe the regulation of fluids and electrolytes by the kidneys.

54.5 Describe the regulation of hydrogen ion balance by the kidneys.

54.6 Describe the regulation of blood pressure by the kidneys.

54.7 Identify other metabolic and endocrine functions of the kidneys.

54.8 Describe the process of micturition.

54.9 Discuss how aging affects urinary function.

Facilitating Student Learning

CLASSROOM

Review Activity

- Give students a nongraded pretest on the basic concepts involved in kidney function.

Class Assignments

- Assign students to complete Chapter 54 in the Study Guide before class.
- Assign selected students to discuss the following concepts in class: glomerular filtration, tubular reabsorption, regulation of fluids and electrolytes by the kidneys, regulation of hydrogen ion balance by the kidneys, and regulation of blood pressure by the kidneys.

Lecture/Discussion

- Ask students to recall from their anatomy and physiology course the functions of the main parts of the urinary system.
- Use the results from the pretest to determine what topics to include in class. Transparencies 105(T) and 106(T) will help stimulate student participation.
- Review with the students how the kidneys rid the blood of waste products and regulate fluid, electrolyte, and acid-base balance. Review urine formation.

Transparencies

- 105(T)—Macroscopic Structure of the Kidney
- 106(T)—Anatomic Relationships of Kidneys and Related Structures

CHAPTER

55

Assessment of Clients with Urinary Disorders

Objectives

55.1 Describe the elements included in a urologic history.

55.2 Describe common urologic symptoms.

55.3 Describe the basic physical examination of clients with urinary disorders.

55.4 Discuss the invasive and noninvasive diagnostic studies used to evaluate urinary function.

55.5 Discuss nursing responsibilities related to selected diagnostic procedures used to evaluate urinary function.

55.6 Recognize abnormal findings in a routine urinalysis.

Facilitating Student Learning

CLASSROOM

Review Activities

- Suggest students review the chapter on urinary elimination in their fundamentals or basic nursing text.
- Suggest students go to the psychomotor skills laboratory for review of the catheterization procedure.

Class Assignments

- Ask students to complete Chapter 55 in the Study Guide before class.
- Ask selected students to present material on invasive methods of monitoring the urinary status, such as intravenous pyelogram, retrograde pyelogram, cystoscopy, and renal biopsy.

Lecture/Discussion

- Demonstrate techniques to be used in collecting a urologic history. Ask another faculty member to role play the client experiencing the urinary disorder. Follow demonstration with a discussion of the physical and psychosocial factors identified by the students.
- Discuss selected diagnostic studies in class. Students can read the material on their own; lecture method will probably not enhance learning of this content.
- Discuss the nurse's role in collecting and testing specimens and assisting the physician in certain diagnostic procedures.
- Encourage students to discuss how the results of diagnostic studies impact the client's plan of care.

Transparencies

- 107(T)—Percussion over the Costovertebral Angle
- 108(T)—Palpating the Kidneys
- 109(T)—Renal Clearance

Guest Speakers

- Invite a radiologist to discuss radiologic studies used to determine urinary function.
- Invite a urology clinical specialist to discuss the nurse's role in preparing clients for diagnostic studies.

CLINICAL

Skills Laboratory

- Discuss techniques used during the physical examination of a client with a urinary disorder. Transparencies 107(T) and 108(T) could be used for clarification.
- Assign pairs of students to practice history-taking and physical examination skills pertinent to assessing persons experiencing urinary disorders. Ask students to document their findings.
- Assign pairs of students to role play teaching and preparing individuals for diagnostic tests; e.g., one student would teach the other student how to collect a clean-catch urine specimen.

Clinical Site Activities

- Evaluate students' history-taking and physical examination skills pertinent to assessing clients with urinary disorders.
- Ask students to correlate the laboratory data (blood chemistry, renal profile, urinalysis, urine culture and sensitivities, etc.) with the client's urinary function.
- Suggest that students review the urine collection procedures for their assigned agency.
- Ask students to assess the urinary status of their assigned client.
- Assign students to clients having diagnostic procedures for assessing urinary function. Arrange for the students to accompany the clients to radiology, clinic, etc., for the procedures. Discuss with individual students their plans for providing care for the clients.

Clinical Conference Activities

- Have students role play giving instructions to clients scheduled for selected diagnostic procedures.
- Ask students to share their experiences in radiology, clinic, etc. Have students identify how these experiences will help them in planning care for such clients in the future.

CHAPTER

56

Nursing Care of Clients with Disorders of the Ureters, Bladder, and Urethra

Objectives

56.1 Describe the etiology and pathophysiology of selected disorders of the ureters, bladder, and urethra, including infections, bladder cancer, urinary tract stones, urinary incontinence, and trauma.

56.2 Summarize the clinical manifestations and medical/surgical management of selected disorders of the ureters, bladder, and urethra.

56.3 Assess clients for clinical manifestations of selected disorders of the ureters, bladder, and urethra.

56.4 Plan individualized nursing interventions for clients with both acute and chronic disorders of the ureters, bladder, and urethra.

56.5 Perform nursing interventions appropriate for clients with urinary tract disorders.

56.6 Evaluate effectiveness of nursing care of clients with urinary tract disorders.

Facilitating Student Learning

CLASSROOM

Review Activity

- Ask students to review the following content found in a fundamentals or basic nursing text: (a) urinary catheterizations, (b) catheter care, (c) bladder irrigation, and (d) applying a condom catheter.

Class Assignments

- Assign students to complete the section in the Study Guide before class session.
- Have students select a urinary tract disorder that they want to study in more depth. Assign students to find two journal articles that address this disorder (one of the articles should be a nursing research study). Ask the students to share their findings with the class.
- Provide the students with a list of diagnostic findings. Ask the students to interpret these values and relate their interpretations to urinary function.

Lecture/Discussion

- This chapter contains information on many important disorders. Review your curriculum to determine if any of these disorders are discussed in other courses. It is recommended that the following disorders be emphasized: urinary tract infection, urinary incontinence, bladder cancer, and neurogenic bladder dysfunction. Other disorders can be covered through the Study Guide or separate study sheets.
- Discuss the potential causes and effects of urinary tract obstruction. Use Transparency 110(T) to clarify content.
- Lead a class discussion to outline the nursing interventions appropriate for the nursing diagnosis Alteration in urinary elimination pattern related to urinary retention.
- Discuss the five major types of neurogenic bladder dysfunction and the resulting problems of urinary elimination. Transparencies 111(T)–115(T) may be used to clarify information.
- Lead a class discussion to outline the nursing interventions appropriate for the nursing diagnosis Alteration in urinary elimination pattern related to urinary incontinence.
- Review how structure and function of the urinary tract changes with age. Discuss the problems of urinary elimination that may result.
- Lead a class discussion to outline the nursing interventions appropriate for the nursing diagnosis Knowledge deficit related to prevention of urinary tract infection.
- Discuss nursing care for clients receiving surgical and nonsurgical management of bladder cancer.
- Lead a class discussion to outline the nursing interventions appropriate for the following three nursing diagnoses: (1) Disturbance in self-concept, body image, and self-esteem related to urinary diversion, (2) Knowledge deficit related to self-care following urinary diversion, and (3) Potential or actual impairment of skin integrity related to urinary diversion.
- Develop a case study of a client coming to a physician's office with bloody urine.

Transparencies

- 110(T)—Potential Effects of Urinary Tract Obstruction
- 111(T)—Neurogenic Bladder Dysfunction: Uninhibited Neurogenic
- 112(T)—Neurogenic Bladder Dysfunction: Sensory Paralytic
- 113(T)—Neurogenic Bladder Dysfunction: Motor
- 114(T)—Neurogenic Bladder Dysfunction: Autonomous
- 115(T)—Neurogenic Bladder Dysfunction: Reflex

Group Activity

- Divide the class into small groups. Ask each group to develop one of the following teaching plans: clients experiencing incontinence, prevention of urinary tract infections, or clients needing to learn intermittent self-catheterization.

Guest Speaker

- Invite an enterostomal therapist to discuss special needs of clients with urinary diversions. Ask the therapist to discuss the specific nursing interventions needed to meet these needs. Suggest that the therapist bring the newest equipment and supplies for stoma care. (Note: If the class is very large, the therapist may be willing to come to clinical conference or lend the equipment and supplies for the students to see during conference.)

CLINICAL

Skills Laboratory

- If needed, assign students to review the skill of urinary catheterization, condom catheters, leg bags, and applying ostomy appliances.
- Demonstrate stoma care on a mannequin and ask students to perform a return demonstration.

Clinical Site Activities

- Assign students to provide care for clients with urinary tract dysfunctions in the urology clinic and on a healthcare facility unit.
- Arrange for students to accompany an enterostomal therapist to learn techniques for providing stoma care for clients with urinary diversions.
- Assign as many students as possible to provide care for clients with urinary diversions.
- Arrange for students to accompany clients undergoing surgery for correction of urinary tract dysfunctions. Ask students to develop a comprehensive care plan for the perioperative period.
- If possible, arrange for selected students to visit the biofeedback laboratory to learn how biofeedback and behavior modification are used in a bladder training program.
- Ask students to correlate medications they give as treatment of urinary tract dysfunction with the client's signs and symptoms and laboratory data; for example, urine culture and sensitivity reports with antibiotic therapy.
- Ask students to review charts of clients hospitalized on their assigned clinical unit to determine the incidence of and contributing factors to nosocomial urinary tract infections.

Clinical Conference Activities

- Invite someone from the Ostomy Association to discuss special needs of an individual with a urinary diversion.
- Invite an ostomy nurse to present an in-service on ostomies. Have the students practice skin care and applying various pouches.
- Consider giving the following extra-credit assignment for theory or clinical: have the students wear an ostomy pouch ⅓-filled with fluid for 24 hours and then write a short paper on the experience. Lead the students in a discussion of the assignment.
- Lead a discussion on students' findings on nosocomial urinary tract infections (see Clinical Site Activities).
- Ask students to give case presentations of the clients for whom they have provided care and to outline the plan of care they used.

Critical Points to Emphasize

Urinary Tract Infection	Bladder Cancer	Urinary Calculi
• Risk factors (Figure 56-1) • Most common nosocomial infection (hospital-acquired) • Gram negative *E. coli* is responsible for approximately 90% of UTIs in women. • Most common clinical manifestations of cystitis • Diagnostic tests • Routine urinalysis and culture and sensitivity; IVP • Rationale for wanting the urine acidic or alkaline • Diets and medications that make the urine acidic (Table 56-2) • Overview of medications to treat cystitis and other urinary disorders (Table 56-1) • Community and self-care • Modifications for elderly clients	• Cardinal sign: painless hematuria • Most frequent cancer in the urinary system • Risk factors (Figure 56-2) • Critical monitoring after urinary diversion procedure (Figure 56-3) • Caring for an ileal conduit at home (Figure 56-3A) • Applying a disposable ostomy pouch (Figure 56-5) • Learning to care for urinary diversion (Figure 56-4) • Importance of self-catheterization for continent pouches	• Risk factors and levels of prevention (Figure 56-5) • Different types of stones especially calcium and uric acid • Reoccurrence rate • Uric acid stones cannot be seen on x-ray. These are diagnosed with history and serum uric acid levels. • Acute medical management: emphasize fluids and ambulation • Stone prevention diet (Figure 56-6) • Strain all urine; when stones are retrieved send to lab to be analyzed

Urinary Incontinence	Urinary Retention	General Information
• Incontinence is involuntary loss of control of voiding. • Types of incontinence (Table 56-3) • Risk factors and levels of prevention (Figure 56-7) • Diagnostic tests: urodynamic studies • Medical management is the major treatment. • AHCPR guidelines • Medications used to treat urge, reflux, and stress incontinence (Table 56-4) • Kegel exercises interesting point: nursing research (Figure 56-8) • Bladder training • Pharmacologic treatment • Bladder retraining • Modifications for elderly clients • Algorithm for urine incontinence (Figure 56-12)	• Primary manifestation is distended bladder and inability to void • Incontinence can also signal retention • BPH the most common cause • Potential effects of urinary obstruction (Figure 56-6) • Medications that cause urinary retention • Major diagnostic test for retention is catheterization. If more than 250–500 mL of urine is in bladder and the client is unable to void, retention is present. • Nursing interventions for voiding • Modifications for elderly clients	• How to assess for bladder distention • Review the catheterization procedure • Nursing care of a client with a Foley catheter • Nursing care of a client with a suprapubic catheter • Which catheters can and cannot be irrigated • How much urine the renal pelvis can hold (5 cc) and the implications • Variations in color of urine • Review routine urinalysis and culture and sensitivity • Modifications for elderly clients

CHAPTER

57

Nursing Care of Clients with Renal Disorders

Objectives

57.1 Describe the etiology, risk factors, and pathophysiology of selected renal disorders.

57.2 Summarize the clinical manifestations, complications, and medical and surgical management of renal disorders.

57.3 Compare and contrast acute and chronic renal failure.

57.4 Plan individualized nursing interventions for clients with renal disorders.

57.5 Evaluate the effectiveness of nursing care of clients with renal disorders.

Facilitating Student Learning

CLASSROOM

Review Activity

- Assign students to review the normal renal anatomy and physiology.

Class Assignments

- Assign students to complete Chapter 57 in the Study Guide before class.
- Assign groups of students to make a list of nephrotoxic drugs using their pharmacology texts as a reference. Each group of students could be responsible for a different classification of pharmacologic agents. Lists could be discussed and shared in class or clinical conference.
- Have students select a urinary tract disorder that they want to study in more depth. Assign students to find two journal articles that address this disorder (one of the articles should be a nursing research study). Ask the students to share findings with the class.
- Provide the students with a list of diagnostic findings. Ask the students to interpret these values and relate their interpretations to renal function.
- Assign students to write a paper on the ethical issues associated with renal dialysis and renal transplant.

Lecture/Discussion

- Briefly discuss the extrarenal conditions and nephrotoxins that can produce renal disorders.
- Discuss various kidney disorders that increase the risk and severity of renal infection. Stress the importance of teaching the client how to decrease the risk of infection.
- Use case presentations to discuss the following kidney disorders: pyelonephritis, glomerulonephritis, nephrotic syndrome, and renal calculi. (Include pathophysiology, usual medical/surgical treatment, nursing diagnoses, and appropriate nursing interventions.)
- Different types of kidney stones obtained from the pathology laboratory and x-rays obtained with intravenous pyelograms of clients with kidney stones make interesting displays when discussing renal calculi.
- Compare and contrast acute and chronic renal failure as to etiology, pathophysiology, clinical course and effects, assessment findings, and interventions.
- Discuss the concept of dialysis. Transparencies 116(T) and 117(T) can be used to clarify content. Provide the students with information on the financial cost for the various methods of dialysis.
- Lead a discussion on the nursing diagnoses and appropriate interventions for clients undergoing dialysis.
- Discuss renal transplantation as an example of organ transplantation. Include the following topics: the guidelines to determine brain death, the general criteria for organ donors, the approximate number of people waiting for kidney transplants, the financial costs, and the legal and ethical issues involved. Up-to-date information may be obtained from the American Council on Transplantation, an organ procurement program, or a transplant center.
- Describe briefly the transplantation procedure. Transparency 118(T) may be used.
- Discuss nursing care for the recipient and donor of a renal transplant.

Transparencies

- 116(T)—Three Types of Peritoneal Dialysis Catheters
- 117(T)—Internal Arteriovenous Fistula
- 118(T)—Transplanted Kidney Placement

Guest Speakers

- Invite a dietitian to discuss nutritional support for persons with the following kidney disorders: renal calculi, nephrotic syndrome, and renal failure.

- Invite a nurse on the transplant team to discuss trends in renal transplantation and organ donation.

CLINICAL

Skills Laboratory

- If possible, set up displays of various pieces of equipment used in peritoneal and hemodialysis.

Clinical Site Activities

- Ask students to explain how the medications they administer are excreted. If the specific drugs are nephrotoxic, ask them what they can do to decrease the risk of renal damage.
- Assign students to clients with various types of kidney disorders. Assist the students as needed in developing nursing care plans.
- Arrange for students to observe the dialysis procedures in the dialysis unit.
- Assign selected students to follow clients as they come to a facility once or twice a week for renal dialysis. After several visits, discuss with the students the particular stresses of these individuals and their significant others. Ask the students to identify the coping mechanisms the clients use.
- Arrange for students to visit clients who use home dialysis. Students would need objectives established before the visit. This assignment could be made in cooperation with community health faculty.
- Arrange for selected students to accompany clients undergoing renal surgery. Ask the students to develop care plans for each phase of the perioperative period.

Clinical Conference Activities

- Ask students to share the nursing care plans they developed. As a group, ask the students to compare and contrast the plans developed for clients with disorders involving inflammation, trauma, infection, lithiasis, or neoplasia.
- Lead a discussion on the ethics involved in renal transplantation.
- Invite a few individuals to conference who have chronic renal disease and have been managed by dialysis or transplantation. Ask them to share their experiences with the students.

CHAPTER

58

Structure and Function of the Gastrointestinal System

Objectives

58.1 Describe the structure and function of the digestive system.

58.2 Describe the normal structure and function of the mouth, esophagus, stomach, and small and large intestines.

58.3 Discuss the effects of aging on the gastrointestinal tract.

Facilitating Student Learning

CLASSROOM

Review Activities

- The objectives listed for Chapter 58 are for review and can be shared with students.
- Assign students to complete the review questions in Chapter 58 the Study Guide. If students are very familiar with the content they will be able to move quickly through the review.

Transparency

- 119(T)—Components of the Gastrointestinal Tract

CHAPTER

59

Assessment of Clients with Gastrointestinal Disorders

OBJECTIVES

59.1 Identify elements of a complete history and physical examination of the gastrointestinal (GI) tract.

59.2 Describe common diagnostic tests used for clients with disorders of the GI system.

Facilitating Student Learning

CLASSROOM

Review Activity

- Review taking a diet history and doing a nutritional assessment (guidelines in Chapter 11).

Lecture/Discussion

- Discuss various diagnostic tests with emphasis on the role of the nurse in preparation of the client for the procedure and any postprocedure nursing care.
- Demonstrate a physical assessment of the GI tract.

Transparency

- 120(T)—Anatomic Regions of the Abdomen

CLINICAL

Skills Laboratory

- Pair students and assign them to do an assessment of the GI system on one another.

Clinical Site Activities

- Assign students to clients with GI disorders and have them collect data on alterations in GI functions.
- Assign students to prepare and accompany clients for various GI studies, or alternatively to spend time in the GI diagnostic laboratory.

Clinical Conference Activity

- Ask students to share their experiences in preparing clients for and accompanying them to various GI procedures.

CHAPTER

60

Nursing Care of Clients with Ingestive Disorders

Objectives

60.1 Discuss disorders associated with the mouth, and medical treatment, associated nursing care, and appropriate primary prevention of these disorders.

60.2 Describe disorders associated with the esophagus, and medical treatment, associated nursing care, and appropriate primary prevention of these disorders.

Facilitating Student Learning

CLASSROOM

Review Activities

- Assign students to review assessment of the oral cavity.
- Review Chapter 58 on structure and function of the oral cavity.
- Review Chapter 59 on assessment of the oral cavity.

Lecture/Discussion

- Discuss the nurse's role in prevention of dental problems, oral cancer, gastroesophageal reflux disease (GERD), and esophageal cancer.
- Obtain slides from an ear, nose, and throat (ENT) specialist that show leukoplakia and oral cancer.
- View an AV on the effects of smokeless tobacco. One suggestion is *Smokeless Tobacco: A New Threat to Public Health*, by K. Thomas Roblins and Alan Blume, Network for Continuing Medical Changes, and Prevention Measures. This film has a medical focus and it includes statistics about smokeless tobacco, cellular changes, and prevention measures.
- Discuss the issues surrounding use of smokeless tobacco.
- Emphasize the role of "healthy teeth" in the maintenance of good nutrition.
- Emphasize the potential effects on the oral cavity when the client is immunosuppressed, and related nursing care.
- Briefly discuss nursing care for the client with oral candidiasis.
- Discuss the safety precautions necessary when a person has dysphagia.
- Discuss the various types of hiatal hernia using Transparency 121(T).
- Discuss nursing care with medical and surgical interventions for hiatal hernia.
- Discuss nursing care for persons with esophageal cancer.
- Discuss client teaching for the person with GERD.
- Discuss nursing care for the client with PEG or PEJ feeding tube.

Transparency

- 121(T)—Hiatal Hernias

CLINICAL

Clinical Site Activities

- Assign students to do a complete oral exam on their assigned clients.
- Have students prepare a teaching module for clients who use smokeless tobacco.
- Assign students to care for persons with disorders of the mouth and/or esophagus.
- Assign students to assess safety precautions being implemented for clients with dysphagia.
- Assign students to review their clinical setting protocols/procedures for PEG or PEJ tube feeding.

Clinical Conference Activities

- Ask students to compare their outcomes on oral assessments.
- Have students who have cared for clients having surgery discuss the rationale for good oral hygiene pre- and postoperatively.

Critical Points to Emphasize

Oral Cancer

- Nurse's role in primary care
- Role of leukoplakia as precancerous lesion
- Causes
- Basal and squamous cell types
- Medical and surgical treatments
- Nursing care: nutrition teaching; pain relief; oral hygiene; teach care, suctioning, emotional support, airway maintenance, prevention of hemorrhage, bed position, and communication techniques

GERD

- Incidence
- Risk factors
- Primary prevention
- Pathophysiology
- Clinical manifestations
- Medical management
- Pharmacologic therapy
- Nursing care: dietary teaching, medications, and lifestyle changes
- Surgical management
- Nursing care: postop care, chest tube maintenance, client teaching, nasogastric (NG) tube maintenance, infection prevention, and nutrition

Candidiasis

- Causes
- Impact in the immunosuppressed client
- Pathophysiology
- Assessment characteristics
- Pharmacologic therapy
- Nursing care: pain relief, nutrition maintenance, use of topical antifungal, client teaching about oral hygiene and not using commercial mouthwash

Hiatal Hernia

- Different types of hiatal hernia
- Pathophysiology
- Clinical manifestations
- Medical and surgical management (see GERD)
- Nursing management (GERD)

CHAPTER

61

Nursing Care of Clients with Gastric Disorders

Objectives

61.1 Identify general clinical manifestations of gastric disorders.

61.2 Discuss types of gastric tubes and care of clients with these tubes.

61.3 Discuss nutritional support for clients with gastric disorders.

61.4 Describe the clinical problems most frequently associated with the stomach and their medical, surgical, and nursing management.

Facilitating Student Learning

CLASSROOM

Review Activities

- Have students review content in Chapter 58 on structure and function of the stomach.
- Suggest that students also review content in Chapter 59 on physical assessment of the abdomen.

Lecture/Discussion

- Discuss the physiologic bases of vomiting and gastric pain.
- Emphasize the medications that are likely to contribute to gastroduodenal ulceration.
- Discuss the nurse's responsibilities when administering total parenteral nutrition and enteral feedings.
- Discuss the pathophysiology and care for persons with eating disorders.
- Discuss development of realistic weight loss goals and interventions for clients who are obese.
- Discuss the pathophysiology and treatment for persons with ulcer disease.
- Explain the physiologic manifestations of dumping syndrome and the rationale for interventions.

Transparencies

- 122(T)—Vagotomy, Pyloroplasty, and Gastroenterostomy
- 123(T)—Insertion of Catheter into Superior Vena Cava Via Right Subclavian Vein
- 124(T)—Total Gastrectomies
- 125(T)—Subtotal Gastrectomies
- 126(T) —Comparison of Peptic Ulcers
- 127(T) —Potential Problems with Total Parenteral Nutrition

CLINICAL

Skills Laboratory

- Work with students in the skills laboratory on changing central line dressing, adding IVs to central lines, and assessing central line sites.
- Work with students on insertion, maintenance, and differentiation of gastrointestinal tubes.

Clinical Site Activities

- Assign students to clients with various types of ulcers and have them identify from client history and physical examination how the person's clinical picture compares to or differs from the textbook picture.
- Assign students to clients who are receiving total parenteral nutrition or enteral feedings. Have them develop care plans that include identification of and treatment for potential problems with these two therapies.

Clinical Conference Activities

- Assign students who have cared for clients with ulcer disease to present their clients in postconference. Have the students compare similarities and differences in client signs and symptoms, history, medical and surgical management, and nursing care.
- Invite group leaders from TOPS, Overeaters Anonymous, and Weight Watchers to describe their programs. Invite a dietitian to give pros and cons of each program and to make additional "realistic" suggestions that students could use when working with clients who are overweight.
- Ask students to discuss their feelings about obese people and behaviors of others in clinical that might indicate a bias against obese people. Have the students discuss approaches they could use that would be nonjudgmental.
- Assign students to identify high-risk clients for stress/drug induced ulcers. Have them also identify assessment items they would include in a nursing care plan when caring for a person at risk.

Critical Points to Emphasize

Parenteral Nutrition

- Examples of clients who may require parenteral nutrition
- Routes
- Solutions
- Complications: insertion, infection, hyper and hypoglycemia, fluid and electrolyte imbalance
- Nursing management: sterile technique with dressing change, equipment, flow rate, assessment, safety

Acute Gastritis

- Etiology
- Risk Factors: Staphylococcus and food substances
- Associated disorders
- Pathophysiology
- Clinical manifestations
- Medical management
- Nursing management: pain control, teaching, medications, NPO with severe nausea and vomiting, fluid and food support

Eating Disorders

- Major disorders
- Pathophysiology
- Clinical Manifestations
- Risk factors
- Medical management
- Nursing management: assistance with selection of foods, monitoring of eating, education, primary prevention, exercise, assessment for electrolyte imbalance and dysrhythmias

Ulcers

- Differentiate types of ulcers
- Etiology
- Risk factors
- Pathophysiology
- Clinical manifestations—comparison of three types
- Medical management: emphasize medications
- Complications
- Nursing management: assessment of lifestyle, physical assessment, pain control, medications, rest, teaching, assessment for complications
- Surgical management
- Nursing management: care of pre- and postoperative client, teaching about postoperative nutritional needs, assessment for postoperative complications, teaching about dumping syndrome

CHAPTER

62

Nursing Care of Clients with Intestinal Disorders

Objectives

62.1 Identify common assessment data for various disorders of the intestinal tract.

62.2 Describe inflammatory disorders of the small and large intestines, medical and surgical management, and nursing care.

62.3 Discuss neoplasms of the intestines, medical and surgical management, and nursing care.

62.4 Describe various ostomy procedures and their nursing management.

62.5 Discuss other disorders of the small and large intestines.

62.6 Describe the effects of blunt or penetrating trauma on the intestines, and medical and nursing management.

62.7 Describe the effects of intestinal obstruction, medical and surgical management, and nursing care.

Facilitating Student Learning

CLASSROOM

Review Activity

- Review standard components of pre- and postoperative nursing care (Chapter 21). Identify any special aspects for clients having surgery on the small or large intestine that need to be added to pre- and postoperative care.

Lecture/Discussion

- Discuss the various bacterial, parasitic infections, and chemical effects on the intestines.
- Compare and contrast Crohn's disease and ulcerative colitis.
- Focus class discussion on nursing care for persons with ostomies. Have students compare and contrast potential problems with the various ostomy procedures.
- Discuss the pathophysiology of, assessment for, and interventions with peritonitis.
- Discuss the components viewed as possible risk factors in the development of colon cancer. Ask students to contribute information they have obtained from the popular media and advertisements.
- Discuss with students the medical, surgical, and nursing management of clients with colon cancer; emphasize aspects of early detection.
- Provide students with a worksheet listing disorders identified in the section of "other disorders of the large and small intestines." Have students define or describe each of the disorders.
- Briefly discuss the effects of blunt or penetrating trauma of the intestines.
- Discuss the effects of obstructions of the large and small intestines.

Transparencies

- 127(T)—The Ileoanal Anastomosis
- 128(T)—The Continent Ileostomy
- 129(T)—Causes of GI Bleeding
- 130(T)—Differentiation of Crohn's Disease and Ulcerative Colitis
- 131(T)—Types of Colostomies

Guest Speakers

- Invite an enterostomal therapist to discuss nursing care of clients with ostomies.
- Invite a member of an ostomy group to discuss the client view of supportive nursing care.

Group Activity

- Assign one group of students to find the American Cancer Society's recommendations for screening for colon cancer. Assign another group of students to talk to a physician with a specialty in gastroenterology to determine his or her recommendations for screening for colon cancer. From the above information have students develop a teaching plan that they could use for all clients, whether in the hospital, clinics, or the community.

CLINICAL

Skills Laboratory

- Assign students to practice applying ostomy pouches, and if mannequins are available, to perform ostomy irrigations.
- Lead a discussion on and demonstrate various approaches to skin care for the client with an ostomy.

Clinical Site Activities

- Assign students to clients with intestinal disorders and have them obtain health histories and do a physical assessment pertinent to the intestinal tract.
- Ask students caring for clients after intestinal surgery to describe when they expect normal bowel sounds to return and explain why bowel sounds are absent in the immediate postsurgical assessment.
- Assign students to accompany the enterostomal therapist for a day to learn about care of clients with ostomies. Suggest that students focus not only on the technical aspects of care but also to observe the therapist's communication techniques and choice of terms when talking about the equipment.

Clinical Conference Activities

- Assign a group of students to develop a teaching plan for colostomy irrigations.
- From their experiences with clients with ostomies and from their readings, have students discuss language that clients with ostomies prefer regarding their equipment.
- Have students discuss activities in which clients with ostomies can participate and those which they might have to restrict.

Critical Points to Emphasize

Gastroenteritis

- Causes with emphasis on hospital acquired *Clostridium difficile*
- Manifestations
- Medical management
- Medications
- Nursing management: assessment of stools, fluid and electrolyte status, comfort measures for skin, medications, and client teaching

Crohn's Disease/Ulcerative Colitis

- Pathophysiology
- Etiology
- Risk factors
- Manifestations/compare and contrast
- Medical management: emphasize medications, use of TPN
- Nursing management: control of diarrhea, nutrition, pain control, coping, referral to Crohn's and Colitis Foundation
- Surgical management: ostomy procedures
- Nursing management: teaching about care of ostomy, pre- and postop care, emotional support, prevention of postop complications

Appendicitis

- Etiology
- Risk factors
- Pathophysiology
- Clinical manifestations
- Surgical management
- Nursing management: assessment, pain control, emphasis on not using laxatives or enemas, NG tube maintenance, assessment for infection, and postoperative care

Colon Cancer

- Etiology
- Early detection guidelines
- Risk factors
- Pathophysiology
- Clinical manifestations
- Diagnostics
- Staging systems
- Medical management
- Nursing management: care of the client receiving radiation and chemotherapy
- Surgical management: types of surgical procedures
- Nursing management: nutrition, bowel preparation, pre- and postop care, emotional support, prevention of postop complications, teaching about care of ostomy

Hernia	Obstruction
• Pathophysiology • Types of hernias • Medical management • Surgical management • Nursing management: pre- and postop care	• Etiology • Pathophysiology • Clinical manifestations • Medical management • Nursing management: fluids and electrolyte imbalance, assessment for shock • Surgical management • Nursing management: pre- and postop care, medications, assessment for complications

CHAPTER

63

Structure and Function of the Liver, Biliary Tract, and Exocrine Pancreas

Objectives

63.1 Describe the normal structure of the liver, biliary tract, and exocrine pancreas.

63.2 Describe the normal function of the liver, biliary tract, and exocrine pancreas.

Facilitating Student Learning

CLASSROOM

Review Activity

- Assign students to answer the study questions in the student study guide. If they are unable to answer the questions, suggest they review the anatomy and physiology of the liver, biliary tract, and pancreas before proceeding to the next chapters.

Transparencies

- 132(T)—Liver Lobules
- 133(T)—Features of the Biliary Tract and Pancreas

CHAPTER

64

Assessment of Clients with Liver, Biliary Tract, and Exocrine Pancreatic Disorders

Objectives

64.1 Prepare a plan for complete assessment of an individual's liver, biliary tract, and pancreatic function.

64.2 Prepare a person with dysfunction of the liver, biliary tract, or pancreas for diagnostic tests.

64.3 Interpret results of laboratory and diagnostic tests.

Facilitating Student Learning

CLASSROOM

Lecture/Discussion

- Emphasize key elements of the history and physical examination related to the liver, biliary systems, and pancreas.
- Discuss laboratory values related to liver, biliary, and pancreatic function, their interpretation, and implications for nursing care.
- Discuss nursing care for clients having various diagnostic procedures related to the liver, biliary tract, and pancreas.
- Emphasize the importance of checking for allergies to iodine preparations when discussing oral cholecystograms and IV cholangiograms.

Transparency

- 134(T)—Assessment for Ascites

CLINICAL

Skills Laboratory

- Pair students and assign them to take a history and do a physical examination to assess the liver, biliary tract, and pancreas.

Clinical Site Activities

- Assign students to care for clients who are having diagnostic procedures of the liver, biliary tract, or pancreas.
- Assign students to develop teaching plans to explain the procedures and nursing care plans to implement other aspects of care for clients having the various procedures.
- Assign students to complete a focused physical assessment of clients with disorders of the liver, biliary system, or pancreas.
- Assign students to examine laboratory reports looking for results of tests of the liver, biliary tract, and pancreatic function and interpret the findings.

CHAPTER

65

Nursing Care of Clients with Liver Disorders

OBJECTIVES

65.1 Discuss the liver disorder jaundice and related medical and nursing management.

65.2 Describe the clinical problems associated with hepatitis and related medical and nursing management.

65.3 Discuss the liver disorder cirrhosis and its medical, surgical, and nursing management.

65.4 Define other hepatic disorders.

65.5 Describe surgical, medical, nursing, and long-term management of the client with a liver transplant.

Facilitating Student Learning

CLASSROOM

Review Activities

- Assign students to review the structure and function of the hepatic system in Chapter 63.
- Assign students to review assessment of the hepatic system in Chapter 64.
- Suggest that students review the formation of bilirubin. Figure 63-7 in Chapter 63 can serve as a guide.

Lecture/Discussion

- Discuss laboratory tests for bilirubin.
- Discuss the causes, distribution, methods of transmission, and incubation periods for hepatitis A, B, C, D, E, and toxic hepatitis.
- Differentiate for students the laboratory tests for hepatitis A and hepatitis B.
- Develop with the students a nursing diagnosis and interventions related to precautions used for persons with hepatitis.
- Discuss common nursing diagnoses and interventions appropriate for persons with hepatitis.
- Examine the complications of hepatitis.
- Focus a student discussion on how to protect the caregiver from contracting hepatitis.
- Explain the pathophysiologic bases for the signs and symptoms of hepatitis.
- Explain what happens to the normal liver lobule architecture in cirrhosis.
- Examine with students the manifestations of cirrhosis and their pathophysiologic bases.
- Discuss the complications of cirrhosis.
- Outline for students the primary nursing diagnoses and interventions that may be common for clients with cirrhosis.
- Use the manifestations of hepatitis and cirrhosis to help students correlate these with functions of the liver.
- Discuss medical and surgical treatment measures for the client with cirrhosis.
- Discuss the course of primary and metastatic liver cancer.
- Discuss ethical issues surrounding transplantation.
- Discuss immediate and long-term care of the client with a liver transplant.

Transparencies

- 134(T)—Assessment for Ascites
- 135(T)—Portacaval Shunt Procedure: Normal and Cavomesenteric
- 136(T)—Portacaval Shunt Procedure: Portacaval Side-to-Side and Portacaval End-to-Side
- 137(T)—Portacaval Shunt Procedure: Central Splenorectal and Distal Splenorectal
- 138(T)—Sengstaken-Blakemore Tube
- 139(T)—LeVeen Peritoneovenous Shunt

CLINICAL

Skills Laboratory

- Pair students and have them practice assessing for ascites.
- Assign students to practice blood and body fluid precautions.

Clinical Site Activities

- Assign students to care for clients with hepatitis, cirrhosis, or other liver disorders.
- Ask students to interpret their clients' laboratory values.
- Question students assigned to clients with hepatitis about the precautions they are taking to protect themselves.
- Ask students to explain the pathophysiologic bases for the data in their physical assessment.

Clinical Conference Activities

- Focus a student discussion on how alcoholism and drug dependence cause and complicate liver disease.
- Assign students who cared for clients with hepatitis and cirrhosis to do a case presentation. Have them present the nursing diagnosis they identified as the main priority. Suggest that the class contribute interventions for the nursing diagnosis and then compare these to the ones the presenters used with their clients.

Critical Points to Emphasize

Jaundice

- Types of jaundice
- Laboratory test for bilirubin
- Medical management
- Nursing management: treatment for pruritus, coping with body image changes, teaching about jaundice, and treatment

Cirrhosis

- Types of cirrhosis
- Primary prevention
- Pathophysiology
- Clinical manifestations
- Medical management
- Nursing management: risk for hemorrhage, nutrition needs, activity intolerance, caution with hepatotoxic medications, client teaching
- Complications of cirrhosis: Portal hypertension, ascites, and hepatic encephalopathy
- With complications review pathophysiology and relationship to normal liver function
- Medical and surgical management of complications
- Nursing care for client with portal hypertension: teaching activities to reduce risk of rupture; assess for hemorrhage; care of client with esophageal balloon: prevent tissue damage, aspiration, and airway obstruction;

(Continued)

Hepatitis

- Differentiate types of hepatitis by etiology, risk factors, and pathophysiology
- Primary prevention
- Clinical manifestations
- Laboratory tests for viral hepatitis
- Medical management
- Complications
- Nursing management: care of client with fatigue, pruritus, nutrition needs, coping, teaching about home care
- Nursing care precautions

(Concluded) assess for development of encephalopathy; postop portosystem shunt: assessment of respiratory, neurologic, renal, and hemodynamic status • Nursing care of the client with ascites: assess for ascites, fluid and electrolyte imbalances, possible fluid restriction, intake and output, daily weight, avoid aspirin, position patient to ease respiratory distress, cough and deep breathe, attention to skin care, and client education • Nursing care of the client with hepatic encephalopathy: protein-reduced diet, assess for gastrointestinal bleeding, prevention of constipation, assess for hypovolemia, assess vital signs, hourly urine output, assess for electrolyte imbalance, administer lactulose and neomycin as ordered, protection of client from injury, assess for changes in level of consciousness	

CHAPTER

66

Nursing Care of Clients with Biliary Tract and Exocrine Pancreatic Disorders

Objectives

66.1 Discuss clinical problems most frequently associated with the gallbladder and biliary tract and their medical, surgical, and nursing management.

66.2 Discuss clinical problems most frequently associated with the exocrine function of the pancreas and their medical, surgical, and nursing management.

Facilitating Student Learning

CLASSROOM

Review Activities

- Assign students to review the structure and exocrine function of the pancreas and the biliary tract in Chapter 63.
- Assign students to review assessment of the exocrine pancreas and biliary tract in Chapter 64.
- Assign students to review care of the perioperative client in Chapter 21.

Lecture/Discussion

- Describe the incidence of and risk factors for gallbladder disease.
- Explain the pathophysiologic basis for the manifestations of gallbladder disease.
- Differentiate among cholelithiasis, cholecystitis, and choledocholithiasis.
- Discuss the medical and surgical treatment for gallbladder disease. Transparency 140(T) showing T-tube placement may be useful in this discussion.
- Discuss the use of meperidine (Demerol) versus morphine for pain in biliary tract and exocrine pancreatic disorders.
- Discuss nursing diagnoses and interventions common in medical and surgical treatment of gallbladder disease.
- Emphasize the reasons for an increased risk for pneumonia with gallbladder and biliary tract surgery. Transparency 141(T) showing the incision line may be helpful.
- Discuss other potential complications with gallbladder surgery.
- Discuss nursing care of the client having laparoscopic cholecystectomy.
- Emphasize aspects of discharge planning for clients having cholecystectomy and laparoscopic cholecystectomy.
- Discuss the causes and incidence of pancreatitis.
- Discuss the manifestations of pancreatitis and their pathophysiologic bases.
- Emphasize the pathophysiologic basis for pain in pancreatitis and the nurse's role in pain management.
- Discuss medical and surgical management of pancreatitis.
- Discuss nursing diagnoses and interventions common in medical and surgical treatments of pancreatitis.
- Discuss the increasing incidence and risk factors of pancreatic cancer.
- Discuss the effect of pancreatic disorders on client nutrition.

Transparencies

- 140(T)—T-Tube Placement
- 141(T)—Cholecystectomy Incision

CLINICAL

Clinical Site Activities

- Assign students to care for clients with various pancreatic or biliary tract disorders.
- As they complete their health assessment on clients, assign students to complete an analysis of a symptom on pain for a client with pancreatitis or cholecystitis or lithiasis.
- Arrange for students to spend time in a pain clinic or with a nurse who specializes in pain management.
- If possible, assign students to care for clients in the preoperative, intraoperative, and postoperative phases of gallbladder surgery (inpatient and outpatient), and develop a nursing care plan that reflects client needs during each of the phases.

Clinical Conference Activities

- Focus student discussion on the use of pharmacologic and nonpharmacologic interventions to manage pain in acute and chronic pancreatitis.

- Have students compare and contrast clients' responses and recovery time with a cholecystectomy versus a laparoscopic cholecystectomy.
- Work with students to develop a discharge plan for clients having gallbladder surgery.
- Assist students to develop a discharge plan for clients having laparoscopic cholecystectomy.
- Review with students the mechanics for teaching and implementing effective lung hygiene.

Critical Points to Emphasize

Cholelithiasis

- Incidence
- Etiology
- Risk factors
- Pathophysiology
- Clinical manifestations
- Diagnostic tests
- Medical management: rationale for use of Demerol
- Nursing management: assessment, pain control, nasogastric suctioning, control of nausea and vomiting, IV fluids, assessment for fluid and electrolyte imbalances, client teaching, safety concerns with retrograde endoscopy procedure, diet teaching
- Surgical management: differentiate various surgical options and use of T-tubes
- Nursing management of surgical client: postop care, emphasis on lung hygiene, support for anxiety, prevention of postop complications, pain control, oral hygiene, client education about home care, care of a client with a T-tube

Cholecystitis

- Definition
- Etiology
- Pathophysiology
- Risk factors
- Clinical manifestations
- Diagnostic tests
- Medical management
- Nursing management: client assessment (see cholelithiasis)
- Surgical management

(Continued)

(Concluded)

Acute Pancreatitis	Chronic Pancreatitis
• Definition • Etiology • Risk factors • Pathophysiology • Clinical manifestations • Diagnostic tests • Medical management: use of analgesics, dietary management • Nursing management: pain management, client support, vital signs, assessment for electrolyte imbalances, assessment for respiratory complications, NPO and nutrition management, client teaching—particularly about dietary restrictions and medications, assisting the client to cope with alcohol abuse • Surgical management alternatives • Nursing management: assessment, preoperative teaching, postoperative care, assessment of tubes and drains, assessment of pancreatic function (endocrine and exocrine), potential need for insulin and/or pancreatic enzymes, client teaching regarding wound care, diet, and medications; diabetes education as appropriate; absolute avoidance of alcohol; follow-up care with home healthcare nurse	• Differentiate from acute • Clinical manifestations • Medical management: diet, elimination of alcohol, pain control, medications • Surgical management: goals, surgical options

CHAPTER

67

Structure and Function of the Endocrine System

Objectives

67.1 Discuss regulation of endocrine activity by the two major endocrine glands, the hypothalamus and the pituitary.

67.2 Define negative feedback systems controlling blood levels of hormones.

67.3 Describe the role of the hypothalamus in endocrine function.

67.4 Identify the major functions of each endocrine gland by giving the action of each hormone produced by the gland.

Facilitating Student Learning

CLASSROOM

Class Assignment

- Assign students to complete the activities in the Study Guide for Chapter 67.

Lecture/Discussion

- Discuss the difference between endocrine and exocrine glands and ask students to give examples of each.
- Review with the class the importance of neuroendocrine control of body functions. Transparency 145(T) may be used.
- Using a diagram of the endocrine system, ask students to name the various endocrine glands, the specific hormones secreted by each gland, and give the action of each hormone. Transparencies 142(T), 143(T), and 145(T) may be used.
- Emphasize the importance of hormones through a review of the characteristics common to all hormones.
- Use the "salt, sugar, sex" analogy to explain the functions of each of the hormones (mineralocorticoids, glucocorticoids, and androgens) secreted by the adrenal cortex. "Salt" for aldosterone because it controls sodium balance, "sugar" for glucocorticoids because they control carbohydrate metabolism, and "sex" for androgens.
- Help students gain an appreciation of the importance of conducting a thorough assessment by discussing how the endocrine system affects all other body systems.

Transparencies

- 142(T)—Endocrine Glands
- 143(T)—The Principal Endocrine Glands and Their Hormones
- 145(T)—The Hypothalamic Pituitary-Adrenal (HPA) Axis

CHAPTER

68

Assessment of Clients with Endocrine Disorders

Objectives

68.1 Discuss how the endocrine system affects every other body system and the resulting variety of manifestations that may occur with endocrine disorders.

68.2 Appreciate the importance of a thorough history and physical examination in the assessment of clients with endocrine disorders.

68.3 Demonstrate correct technique for palpation of the thyroid gland.

68.4 Identify common diagnostic tests for thyroid, adrenal, and posterior pituitary function.

Facilitating Student Learning

CLASSROOM

Class Assignments

- Assign students to complete the activities in the Study Guide for Chapter 68.
- Assign students to study the overview of nursing assessment of the endocrine system in Chapter 68 of the text. Ask them to determine if there is any body system that is not affected by endocrine disorders.

Lecture/Discussion

- Help students gain an appreciation of the importance of conducting a thorough assessment by discussing how the endocrine system affects all other body systems.
- Present an overview of the most common diagnostic tests for thyroid function (serum$_3$, T_4, and TSH), adrenal function (serum cortisol level, 24-hour urine ketosteroid level, and urine catecholamines and VMA levels), and posterior pituitary function (urine specific gravity, serum osmolarity).

CLINICAL

Skills Laboratory

- Assign groups of students (three in each group) to practice assessment skills with students taking turns being interviewer/ examiner, client, and evaluator.
- Assist students as they practice palpation of the thyroid gland.

Clinical Site Activity

- Assign students to clients with endocrine problems and check their assessment knowledge and skills.

CHAPTER

69

Nursing Care of Clients with Endocrine Disorders of the Pancreas

Objectives

69.1 Discuss current knowledge regarding the etiology of diabetes mellitus.

69.2 Describe the effect of diabetes mellitus on carbohydrate, fat, and protein metabolism.

69.3 List the cardinal symptoms of diabetes mellitus and give the pathophysiologic basis for each.

69.4 Compare and contrast two common types of diabetes mellitus: insulin-dependent and non-insulin–dependent.

69.5 Discuss methods of early detection and assessment factors used in screening and diagnosis of diabetes mellitus.

69.6 Discuss the goal of care for clients with diabetes mellitus and include the criteria for "good control."

69.7 Teach the client the importance of balancing diet, exercise, and rest in order to control or regulate blood glucose levels.

(Continued)

(Concluded)

69.8 State the action, side effects, and nursing implications for insulin and oral hypoglycemic agents.

69.9 List the nursing diagnoses, with rationale and intervention, commonly indicated with diabetes mellitus.

69.10 Differentiate between the pathophysiologies of diabetic ketoacidosis and hyperglycemic, hyperosmolar, nonketotic coma.

69.11 Describe clinical manifestations, diagnostic findings, and management for each of the acute complications listed in Objective 10.

69.12 Differentiate among the long-term complications of diabetes mellitus regarding reversible and irreversible changes.

69.13 Identify the nurse's role in preventing long-term complications for a client with diabetes mellitus.

69.14 Explain the need for the special perioperative care necessary for a client with diabetes mellitus.

Facilitating Student Learning

CLASSROOM

Class Assignments

- Assign students to complete the activities in the Study Guide for Chapter 69.
- Assign students to list the subjects addressed in any recent issue of *Diabetes Care*, a publication of the American Diabetes Association, Inc., and to write a brief review of one article.
- Ask students to develop a care plan for a client with insulin-dependent diabetes mellitus. Various aspects of care may include the following: insulin or hypoglycemic therapy, diet, urine and blood testing, routine health exams, and treatment for any complications.

Lecture/Discussion

- Emphasize that diabetes mellitus is not only "sugar diabetes," but that diabetes mellitus affects protein and fat metabolism. Review the normal effects of insulin: allows transport of glucose into the cell, stimulates protein synthesis, inhibits triglyceride breakdown in the cell, and promotes fatty acid storage.
- Discuss current knowledge regarding the etiology of diabetes mellitus. Include predisposing factors of heredity and obesity, possible precipitating factors of viral illness followed by autoimmune reaction, and the role of receptor sites for insulin.
- Discuss the characteristics of the two common types of diabetes mellitus. Refer students to Tables 69–1 "Selected Clinical Manifestations of Diabetes Mellitus at Diagnosis," and 69–2 "Distinguishing Features of Type I and Type II Diabetes Mellitus" in Chapter 69 of the text.
- Discuss the pharmacologic treatment of diabetes mellitus with insulin and oral hypoglycemics. Include the general characteristics of insulin: onset, peak, and duration of action of the different types with an emphasis on the time of day of peak action because this is when the hypoglycemic reaction is most likely to occur; the Somogyi, or rebound, effect; and complications of insulin therapy. Table 69–5 "Oral Hypoglycemic Agents," Table 69–6 "Types of Human Insulin and Comparative Actions," and Table 69–9 "Interventions for Hypoglycemia" in Chapter 69 of the text, and the activity "Review of Insulin and Oral Hypoglycemics" in the Study Guide for this chapter may be used. Transparency 144(T) may be used when discussing insulin injection sites.
- Compare and contrast diabetic coma (ketoacidosis) and hyperglycemic, hyperosmolar, nonketotic coma (HHNK) as to pathophysiology, usual signs and symptoms, and interventions. Table 69–10 in Chapter 69 of the text may be used.
- Stress the importance of immediate intervention when a hypoglycemic reaction is suspected.
- Explain that brain cells can use glucose without insulin and the administration of carbohydrates is essential to prevent brain damage, myocardial ischemia, extension of a myocardial infarction, or death.
- Discuss the clinical presentation of a person with a hypoglycemic reaction.
- Stress the importance of subjective data in assessing a client for possible hypoglycemia; for instance, if a client says "I feel like my blood sugar is low" or "I need some sugar now," the client is most likely hypoglycemic and should be treated as such.
- Discuss treatment for hypoglycemia for the conscious and unconscious client.
- Discuss the long-term complications of diabetes mellitus with emphasis on methods of early diagnosis and interventions aimed at prevention. Refer students to Table 69–11 in Chapter 69 of the text.

Transparency

- 144(T)—Insulin Injection Sites

Guest Speaker

- A representative from the local chapter of the American Diabetes Association and a clinical nurse specialist or nurse practitioner working with these programs could facilitate the discussion of the nurse's role in mass screening, early detection, and public education programs to identify and assist people with diabetes mellitus.

GROUP ACTIVITIES

- Divide the class into small groups. Assign each group to gather enough nutritional information on foods served at a fast food restaurant to be able to use those foods as substitutes in an ADA diet. Discuss the findings in class.
- Provide students with a case study of a client with insulin-dependent diabetes mellitus. Include the individualized plan for diet, exercise, and insulin. For each group of students, change different factors that could affect the control and ask the students to determine the effects on the client's blood glucose level and the resulting signs and symptoms.

CLINICAL

SKILLS LABORATORY

- Assign students to test their own urine samples for glucose and ketones using various testing methods. Have other urine samples with added glucose and acetone available for the students to use in testing.
- Assign students to test their own blood glucose levels from a finger stick specimen using the Dextrostix and a glucometer if available.
- If students have not gained sufficient practice in giving subcutaneous injections, allow them to give injections of normal saline to each other.
- Show the students how to record the medication administration on an insulin injection record that indicates site, time, and amount and type of insulin.
- Require the students to demonstrate the proper method of mixing NPH and regular insulin in one syringe.
- Assign students to give foot care to each other. This should include a thorough inspection, a focused interview, and a demonstration of proper foot care. The Study Guide activity "Review of Foot Care" in Chapter 69 and the Care Plan in Chapter 69 of the text may be used.

CLINICAL SITE ACTIVITIES

- In the acute care setting, assign each student to at least one client with insulin-dependent diabetes mellitus and one with non-insulin–dependent diabetes mellitus. Focus the students' attention on preventing acute complications as the blood glucose level is being controlled.
- Either in the ambulatory care clinic or in community health, assign each student to a client with diabetes mellitus. Focus the students' attention on helping clients with diabetes mellitus manage self-care.
- If possible, assign each student to a client with diabetes mellitus who also is having surgery. Focus the students' attention on the special care required to prevent complications that may result because of the diabetes.
- Encourage students to participate as volunteers in screening programs for diabetes mellitus.
- Assign students to locate or develop teaching plans for use in their clinical setting to teach self-care to clients with diabetes mellitus.

CLINICAL CONFERENCE ACTIVITIES

- Ask students to share their experiences of caring for clients with diabetes mellitus. Emphasize that diabetes mellitus affects persons they will encounter in every specialty of nursing.
- Invite persons with diabetes mellitus to discuss how they cope with living with the diabetes.
- Invite a representative from the local affiliate of the American Diabetes Association to discuss their work and resources available.
- Discuss ways to help a legally blind person with insulin-dependent diabetes mellitus learn self-care. A clinical nurse specialist who works with clients with diabetes may help. Resource materials are available through the Society for the Blind.
- Invite a nurse who assists clients who are new users of the portable insulin pumps or a person who has adjusted to using the insulin pump, after taking insulin by subcutaneous injections, to discuss the use of the pump.

CHAPTER

70

Nursing Care of Clients with Thyroid and Parathyroid Disorders

OBJECTIVES

70.1 Describe three types of thyroid enlargement (goiter, thyroiditis, and thyroid tumors), giving definition, assessment and methods of diagnosis, and interventions.

70.2 Identify two major forms of hypothyroidism.

70.3 Discuss the etiology of hypothyroidism in adults.

70.4 Discuss the etiology of Graves' disease as an autoimmune disorder.

70.5 Compare and contrast the signs and symptoms of hypo- and hyperthyroidism.

70.6 Describe the complications of hypo- and hyperthyroidism.

70.7 Discuss the usual medical treatment for hypo- and hyperthyroidism.

70.8 Discuss nursing responsibilities regarding thyroid function tests.

70.9 Describe the needs of clients experiencing hypo- and hyperthyroid function.

(Continued)

(Concluded)

70.10 Plan nursing care interventions to meet the needs of clients experiencing hypo- and hyperthyroid function.

70.11 Recognize the signs of under- and overdose of thyroid hormones.

70.12 Give the action and toxic or side effects of antithyroid medications.

70.13 Discuss nursing care for a person receiving radioactive iodine (^{131}I) therapy.

70.14 Discuss types of thyroid cancer as to incidence, characteristics, intervention, and prognosis.

70.15 Discuss nursing care needed to help assure that the client scheduled for a thyroidectomy is euthyroid, relaxed, well-nourished, and has no uncontrolled cardiac problems.

70.16 Describe nursing assessment needed to recognize early signs and symptoms of the major complications that may follow a thyroidectomy.

70.17 Plan postoperative nursing care to decrease strain on the suture line, relieve discomfort from sore throat and tracheal irritation, prevent pooling of respiratory secretions, and prevent or relieve the complications of thyroidectomy.

70.18 Describe hypo- and hyperparathyroidism as to etiology, assessment and methods of diagnosis, and interventions.

70.19 Discuss specifically the treatment of hypercalcemia.

70.20 List nursing diagnoses that may apply to clients experiencing parathyroid disorders.

70.21 Plan nursing interventions based on the list of nursing diagnoses.

70.22 Discuss nursing care needed to meet the goals of preoperative care for a client having a parathyroidectomy.

70.23 Describe nursing assessments needed to recognize early signs and symptoms of the major complications that may follow parathyroid resection.

70.24 Plan postoperative nursing care for clients undergoing parathyroid gland resection.

Facilitating Student Learning

CLASSROOM

Class Assignments

- Assign students to complete the activities in the Study Guide for Chapter 70.
- Ask students to outline nursing interventions for clients experiencing hypo- and hyperthyroidism and hypo- and hyperparathyroidism based on the nursing diagnoses given in the text, and to bring their outlines to class for discussion.

Lecture/Discussion

- Discuss nursing responsibilities regarding thyroid function studies. Table 70–2 in the text may be used.
- Show slides depicting people with various disorders of the thyroid gland. If possible, show companion slides of the people after treatment. Discuss how body image may be affected. Figures 70–1, 70–2, and 70–3 in the text may be used.
- List the nursing diagnoses that may apply to clients experiencing thyroid gland dysfunction, and outline nursing care plans based on those diagnoses, asking the students for suggestions.
- Discuss emergency interventions necessary for a client experiencing thyroid storm (thyrotoxicosis).
- Relate normal function of the parathyroid glands to the signs and symptoms resulting from hypo- and hyperparathyroidism.
- Discuss nursing assessment needed to detect signs and symptoms of hypocalcemic tetany. Transparency 5(T) may be used.
- Stress the importance of teaching people who will be taking medications for treatment of thyroid or parathyroid dysfunction. Tables 70–3 and 70–8, and the Client Education Guide on Thyroid Supplements in the text may be used.

Transparency

- 5(T)—Chvostek's and Trousseau's Signs

CLINICAL

Skills Laboratory

- Ask students to demonstrate physical assessment skills for detecting hypocalcemia: Chvostek's and Trousseau's signs. Emphasize that these signs may not be positive in all cases of hypocalcemia but that they are useful tests. Discuss how they may also use deep tendon reflexes to test for hypocalcemia.
- Assign small groups of students to prepare the bedside environment for a person returning from the recovery room after a thyroidectomy.

Clinical Site Activities

- Assign students to care for persons undergoing either a thyroidectomy or parathyroid gland resection. Preferably, the student should provide care for the person in all phases of the perioperative period.
- Assign students to the endocrinology clinic to observe how persons are given initial diagnostic testing, and how others already diagnosed with thyroid and parathyroid dysfunction are given ongoing treatment and counseling. A nurse practitioner or clinical nurse specialist could assist with the students' learning in this area.

Clinical Conference Activities

- Invite a person who is recovering from a thyroid disorder to discuss how the disorder affected their life and significant others.
- Ask students who have been assigned to care for persons with either thyroid or parathyroid dysfunction to participate in a care planning conference. Students should be prepared to present the "textbook picture" (pathophysiology, usual signs and symptoms, diagnostic tests, and expected nursing diagnoses and interventions), and compare that with similar data regarding the persons for whom they are providing care. Other students could be asked to add their suggestions.

CHAPTER

71

Nursing Care of Clients with Adrenal, Pituitary, and Gonadal Disorders

Objectives

71.1 Compare and contrast the signs and symptoms of adrenocortical insufficiency and adrenocortical hyperfunction.

71.2 Relate the signs and symptoms of Addison's disease to a decrease in production of each of the three groups of adrenocortical hormones.

71.3 Identify four conditions that may cause secondary adrenocortical insufficiency.

71.4 Discuss the danger of acute adrenal insufficiency (Addisonian crisis).

71.5 Describe three types of adrenocortical hyperfunction (Cushing's syndrome, Conn's syndrome, and adrenogenital syndrome) as to definition, etiology, assessment and methods of diagnosis, and interventions.

71.6 Describe the adrenomedullary disorder of pheochromocytoma as to pathophysiology, usual signs and symptoms, methods of diagnosis, and interventions.

(Continued)

(Continued)

71.7 Discuss nursing responsibilities regarding laboratory diagnostic tests to detect specific dysfunctions of the adrenal glands.

71.8 Identify nursing diagnoses based on the needs of clients experiencing dysfunction of the adrenal glands.

71.9 Plan nursing interventions that will decrease the risk of acute paroxysmal hypertension preoperatively and profound shock postoperatively for a person undergoing surgical excision of a pheochromocytoma.

71.10 Recognize the signs of under- and overdosage of corticosteroids.

71.11 Develop a teaching plan for helping a person learn self-administration of steroids.

71.12 List nursing interventions, with rationale for each action, necessary for a person experiencing Addisonian crisis.

71.13 Summarize the pre- and postoperative nursing care of clients undergoing unilateral or bilateral adrenalectomy.

71.14 Describe hyperpituitarism and hypopituitarism as to etiology, assessment and diagnostic methods, and interventions.

71.15 Compare and contrast the signs and symptoms of diabetes insipidus with the syndrome of inappropriate antidiuretic hormone (SIADH).

71.16 Describe diabetes insipidus and SIADH as to etiology, assessment and diagnostic methods, and interventions.

71.17 Discuss teaching needed by the person who is to undergo surgical removal of the pituitary.

71.18 Describe a focused but thorough nurse's assessment of the person prior to surgical removal of the pituitary.

71.19 Differentiate between nursing assessment and intervention following hypophysectomy via a craniotomy and via the transsphenoidal approach.

Facilitating Student Learning

CLASSROOM

CLASS ASSIGNMENTS

- Assign students to complete the activities in the Study Guide for Chapter 71.
- Ask students to study the content on glucocorticoids and mineralocorticoids in a pharmacology text.
- Ask students to review the content on sodium- and potassium-restricted diets in their nutrition text and to describe which dietary modifications might be necessary for clients with either Addison's disease or Cushing's syndrome.

LECTURE/DISCUSSION

- Show slides depicting people with acromegaly. Also show slides depicting people with Cushing's syndrome before and after interventions and refer students to Figure 71–2 in Chapter 71 of the text. Discuss the impact of body image changes and ways to support the client and their significant others.
- Discuss nursing responsibilities in collecting specimens for laboratory tests as a method to diagnose adrenal and pituitary dysfunction. A laboratory technologist could be invited to contribute the following types of information: the cost of the tests, the importance of accurate preparation (for example, dietary restrictions for urinary VMA levels), a complete specimen (for example, 24-hour urine specimens for catecholamine assays). Refer students to Table 71–2 in the text.
- Discuss the major adrenocortical medications by comparing each to cortisone: 25 mg cortisone is equivalent to 5 mg prednisolone, 5 mg prednisone, and 20 mg hydrocortisone. Refer students to Table 71–3 in Chapter 71 of the text.
- Stress the importance of teaching the person about replacement hormonal therapy.
- Give brief case presentations of clients with hypo- and hyperfunction of the adrenal cortex and pituitary gland (anterior and posterior parts). Lead the class in listing the nursing diagnoses and interventions pertinent for each case. Students should bring their completed activity "Care Plan for a Client with Addison's Disease" from the Study Guide to the class discussion.
- Help students understand the pathophysiology of SIADH by explaining the relationship of ADH and aldosterone; for example, serum sodium level decreases and urine sodium level increases because ADH is being released without a feedback mechanism to stop it. Thus, water is retained which decreases the secretion of aldosterone from the adrenal cortex. With decreased levels of aldosterone, the kidney tubules retain less sodium.
- Stress the importance of quick and accurate assessment and intervention for clients experiencing Addisonian crisis, uncontrolled or uncompensated diabetes insipidus, or SIADH.

CLINICAL

SKILLS LABORATORY

- Assign students to check the specific gravity of their urine and to determine possible reasons for the variations.

CLINICAL SITE ACTIVITIES

- Assign students to the endocrinology clinic to observe management of endocrine dysfunction.
- Assign students to care for clients undergoing either an adrenalectomy or hypophysectomy.

CLINICAL CONFERENCE ACTIVITIES

- Ask students to share their clinical site experiences with the group.
- Invite a member of Little People of America to tell how one adapts to a world geared for larger persons.
- Invite a pharmacologist to present pertinent information on steroids. Then, ask the students to develop a teaching plan for a person receiving a steroid replacement.

CHAPTER

72

Structure and Function of the Musculoskeletal System

OBJECTIVES

72.1 Identify parts of the axial and appendicular skeleton.

72.2 Describe the general structure of bone.

72.3 Describe bone classification according to shape.

72.4 Identify five major functions of the skeletal system.

72.5 Describe joint categorization according to the degree of movement.

72.6 Identify movements possible for synovial joints.

72.7 Describe three types of muscles.

72.8 Discuss briefly the physiology of the muscular system to include muscle tone and oxygenation.

72.9 Discuss briefly bone remodeling and bone repair.

Facilitating Student Learning

CLASSROOM

Review Activity

- Ask students to review musculoskeletal structure and function in their anatomy and physiology text.

Class Assignment

- Assign students to complete the activities in the Study Guide for this chapter.

Lecture/Discussion

- For review, conduct a question and answer session on the major points related to structure and function of the musculoskeletal system.

Transparencies

- 146(T)—Divisions of the Skeleton
- 147(T)—Types of Freely Moveable Joints

CLINICAL

Skills Laboratory

- Assign pairs of students to practice passive range of motion exercises and name each movement possible for synovial joints.

CHAPTER

73

Assessment of Clients with Musculoskeletal Disorders

Objectives

73.1 Collect pertinent health history and subjective data regarding symptoms related to musculoskeletal problems.

73.2 Obtain objective data in a systematic manner for a general and focal musculoskeletal assessment.

73.3 Describe neurologic assessment of the peroneal, tibial, radial, ulnar, and median nerves.

73.4 Describe the types and degrees of range of motion possible with each joint.

73.5 Provide information about the following diagnostic procedures to the clients having the procedures: x-rays, tomography, dural-energy x-ray absorptiometry, arthrogram, bone scans, indium imaging, biopsy, arthroscopy, and electromyography.

73.6 Describe nursing interventions specific to pre- and postprocedure care for the following diagnostic procedures: bone or muscle biopsy, arthroscopy, arthrocentesis, and electromyography.

Facilitating Student Learning

CLASSROOM

Review Activity

- Suggest that students review "Musculoskeletal Assessment" in their physical assessment text or on a videotape.

Class Assignment

- Assign students to complete the activities in the Study Guide for this chapter.

Lecture/Discussion

- Review with students the basics of a musculoskeletal assessment. Transparencies 148(T), 149(T), 150(T), and 151(T) may be used.
- Stress the importance of peripheral nerve assessment as part of neurovascular checks for patients with injuries to their extremities. Refer students to Figure 73–6 in Chapter 73 of the text.
- Refer students to Table 73–4, "Common Laboratory Studies Used in Diagnosing Musculoskeletal Conditions" in the text to use as a reference as they study rheumatoid diseases, osteoporosis, bone cancer, and muscular dystrophy.
- Discuss the nurse's role in helping clients having diagnostic procedures to detect or evaluate musculoskeletal problems. Transparency 152(T) may be used.

Transparencies

- 148(T)— Assessing Muscle Strength
- 149(T)—Joint Range of Motion
- 150(T)—Use of Goniometer
- 151(T)—Musculoskeletal Deformities
- 152(M)—Arthroscope Inserted in Knee

CLINICAL

Skills Laboratory

- Assign students to complete an assessment of the musculoskeletal system on each other. Tell them to use the "Neurovascular Assessment Checklist" in the Study Guide.
- Ask students to use Table 73–2, "Joint Function" in the text and perform appropriate tests on their lab partner to assess for the following abnormalities: rotator cuff tear, tennis elbow, carpal tunnel syndrome, ruptured disc, anterior cruciate ligament injury, and meniscus injury.

Clinical Site Activity

- Assign students to an orthopedic clinic to learn assessment of clients with musculoskeletal disorders.

Clinical Conference Activity

- Ask students to identify common problems and nursing diagnoses they encountered in clinical care.

CHAPTER

74

Nursing Care of Clients with Musculoskeletal Disorders

OBJECTIVES

74.1 Compare and contrast the pathophysiology of osteoporosis, Paget's disease, and osteomalacia.

74.2 Discuss risk factors for osteoporosis and preventive measures.

74.3 Describe diagnostic assessment and treatment including discharge teaching for osteoporosis.

74.4 Identify drug therapy for Paget's disease.

74.5 Describe pain and orthopedic complications that may occur with Paget's disease.

74.6 Describe dietary supplements as an intervention for osteomalacia.

74.7 Compare and contrast the etiology and pathophysiology of osteoarthritis and gouty arthritis.

74.8 Describe the main clinical manifestations and diagnostic findings for osteoarthritis and gouty arthritis.

74.9 Identify medical treatment for osteoarthritis and gouty arthritis.

(Continued)

(Concluded)

74.10 Discuss surgical management of the client with arthritis to include indications, techniques, and complications.

74.11 Describe nursing management for the client having a total knee replacement.

74.12 Describe nursing management for the client having a total hip replacement.

74.13 Describe adult scoliosis and surgical management.

74.14 Describe the etiology, diagnosis, and management of osteomyelitis.

74.15 Differentiate between the terms for benign and malignant bone tumors.

74.16 Describe in general terms for the diagnosis and treatment of bone tumors.

74.17 Describe the following common hand and foot disorders as to definition, assessment findings, and treatment: carpal tunnel syndrome, Dupuytren's contracture, ganglion, hallux valgus, hammer toe, and Morton's neuroma.

Facilitating Student Learning

CLASSROOM

Class Assignments

- Divide the class into thirds to do literature reviews from the latest publications on one of the following three topics: 1) current research in the area of malignant bone tumors, 2) recent recommendations for the treatment and prevention of osteoporosis, and 3) development of improved methods of diagnosing and treating scoliosis. Ask students to be prepared to share their findings in class or clinical conference.
- Assign students to complete the activities in the Study Guide for this chapter.

Lecture/Discussion

- Discuss osteoporosis and emphasize the need for prevention through diet, exercise, and calcium supplements. Include the latest in diagnostic techniques, such as the use of dual-energy x-ray absorptiometry and the World Health Organization (WHO) diagnostic categories.
- Discuss osteomyelitis and stress the importance of prevention and early detection if infection should occur so chronic osteomyelitis may be prevented. Discuss medical treatment with intravenous antibiotics and surgical intervention.
- Discuss scoliosis and the need for screening programs and early detection in children and early teens to prevent severe scoliosis in adults.

Transparency

- 162(T)—Osteoporotic Changes

Guest Speakers

- Invite an orthopedic surgeon to discuss the latest developments in surgical treatment of scoliosis.
- Invite a dietitian to discuss dietary recommendations for preventing osteoporosis.

CLINICAL

Clinical Site Activities

- Assign students in the acute care setting to provide care for clients with the various musculoskeletal disorders discussed in class. Expect the students to individualize the standardized care plans and to consider the person's home environment.
- Arrange for students to spend some time in the orthopedic clinics where clients with the various musculoskeletal disorders are seen.

Clinical Conference Activities

- Discuss how alterations in body image (for example, with scoliosis) can affect persons with musculoskeletal disorders and nursing interventions that may be helpful.
- Ask students to share findings from their literature reviews.
- Ask students to share how they needed to individualize standardized care plans.

CHAPTER

75

Nursing Care of Clients with Musculoskeletal Trauma or Overuse

OBJECTIVES

75.1 Identify common types of fractures from a diagram or descriptions.

75.2 Identify signs and symptoms indicative of a fracture.

75.3 Describe the stages of fracture healing.

75.4 Discuss first aid for clients with fractures.

75.5 List the primary goals of treatment for a client with a fracture.

75.6 Describe three basic methods of reducing a fracture.

75.7 Describe the purposes of various types of traction.

75.8 Discuss nursing interventions for clients in traction.

75.9 Discuss potential complications of fractures and give the interventions useful in preventing each complication.

75.10 Describe the purposes of various types of casts.

75.11 Assist with the application and removal of a cast.

(Continued)

(Concluded)

75.12 Discuss nursing interventions for clients with casts.

75.13 Discuss nursing care for the client with a fracture treated with external fixation.

75.14 Describe the types of "hip fractures" (fractures of the proximal end of the femur).

75.15 Identify usual signs and symptoms of a fractured hip.

75.16 Describe potential complications of proximal femur fractures.

75.17 Plan nursing interventions for the client who has undergone surgery to repair a hip fracture.

75.18 Discuss the incidence and type of injuries resulting from sport injuries.

75.19 Describe specific ways to minimize the risk for overuse injuries.

75.20 Discuss common overuse sport injuries as to cause, assessment, and intervention.

75.21 Discuss the goals of physical therapy for clients with musculoskeletal impairment.

75.22 Discuss the application of heat and cold, and the use of massage and exercise.

75.23 Discuss the use of the following assistive devices: crutches, canes, walkers, and supports.

Facilitating Student Learning

CLASSROOM

Review Activity

- Ask students to use their fundamentals or basic nursing text to review the following common interventions for clients experiencing musculoskeletal impairment: the therapeutic application of heat and cold; the use of massage; crutch selection, fitting, and use; and nursing measures to prevent complications of immobility.

Class Assignments

- Suggest that students visit the library to find the number of journals devoted to sports medicine and physical fitness so they might better appreciate the public's need for help in preventing injuries while participating in fitness programs.
- Assign students to complete the Study Guide activities for this chapter.

Lecture/Discussion

- Discuss the purposes of common interventions such as rest, physical therapy, assistive devices, casts, and traction. Discuss the nursing responsibilities involved with each intervention, and stress the importance of preventing complications.
- Discuss opportunities for nurses in physical fitness and wellness programs.
- Discuss assessment, pathology, and interventions for overuse injuries; and emphasize the importance of preventing such injuries.
- Discuss specific musculoskeletal injuries as to usual cause, presenting signs and symptoms, potential complications, and interventions. Transparencies listed below may be used. X-rays depicting various fractures and internal fixation devices make excellent visual aids.
- Discuss the financial costs of musculoskeletal injuries that result in long-term disabilities.
- Discuss nursing diagnoses and appropriate interventions for each diagnosis applicable for clients following hip surgery.

Transparencies

- 153(T)—Buck's Traction
- 154(T)—Russell's Traction
- 155(T)—Head Halter Traction
- 156(T)—Pelvic Traction
- 157(T)—Balanced Suspension Traction
- 158(M)—Skeletal Traction (Courtesy of Zimmer, Inc.)
- 159(M)—Potential Pressure Points with Cast
- 160(M)—Cast Removal
- 161(M)—Crutches
- 163(T)—Sprain Injuries
- 164(M)—Hip Joint Injuries
- 165(M)—Types of Fractures
- 166(T)—Stages of Fracture Healing
- 167(T)—Hip Fractures
- 168(T)—Reduction of Fractures

Guest Speakers

- Invite a nurse from the emergency department and an emergency medical technician to discuss first aid and emergency treatment for clients with musculoskeletal injuries.
- Invite a physician who specializes in sports medicine to discuss this area of healthcare.
- Invite an orthopedic clinical nurse specialist or nurse practitioner to discuss advanced treatment of musculoskeletal injuries, such as external fixation devices and bone grafting.
- Invite an orthopedic clinical nurse specialist, nurse practitioner, or technician to demonstrate various types of traction, and the application and removal of a cast. (If the class is very large, this activity may be used in a skills laboratory.)

Group Activities

- Ask groups of students to identify a specific musculoskeletal injury prevalent among a particular population (such as hip fractures among elderly women) and to develop a teaching plan or public education program aimed at prevention.
- Assign groups of students to develop teaching plans for clients who will be caring for themselves when using the following common interventions used in the management of musculoskeletal impairment: application of heat, application of cold, active exercises, various assistive devices, casts, and intermittent skin traction.

CLINICAL

Skills Laboratory

- Ask students to demonstrate stretching exercises designed to increase muscle flexibility.
- Assign pairs of students to use each other as models to demonstrate assessment for musculoskeletal trauma.
- Ask students to demonstrate back strengthening exercises and correct lifting techniques.
- Assign pairs of students to use each other as models to demonstrate first aid for fractures.
- Demonstrate how to position and turn a client postoperatively following hip surgery, then ask students to give a return demonstration.
- Assign pairs of students to practice giving each other massages and passive exercises.
- Assign pairs of students to fit each other for crutches.
- Assign students to use crutches, a cane, and a walker. Be sure students practice going up and down stairs with the cane and crutches, and use various crutch walking gaits.
- Assign students to practice neurovascular assessment on each other. They may use the "Neurovascular Assessment Checklist" provided in the Study Guide to record their findings.
- Arrange for a class demonstration of cast application and removal, and setting up various types of traction. Ask students to demonstrate the application of Buck's traction, pelvic traction with the bed in Williams' position, and balanced suspension. Review nursing interventions designed to prevent potential complications.

Clinical Site Activities

- Assign students to the orthopedic clinic or emergency department to learn assessment and intervention for clients with musculoskeletal injuries that can be treated in the outpatient setting.
- Assign students to provide care for clients with musculoskeletal injuries treated with traction, or open reduction and internal fixation. Arrange for the students to accompany their clients to the operating and recovery rooms. Ask students to prepare care plans designed to prevent potential complications.
- Arrange for students to visit the physical therapy department to observe physical therapy techniques used for musculoskeletal problems.
- Arrange for students to spend some time in the orthopedic clinic to assist with cast application and to learn nursing interventions helpful in discharge teaching.
- Assign students to provide nursing care for clients in casts or traction. Expect students to include interventions designed to prevent potential complications.

Clinical Conference Activities

- Ask students to compare their care plans designed to prevent potential complications.
- Encourage students to express their feelings about providing nursing care for clients with chronic low back pain.
- Ask students to identify common problems and nursing diagnoses they encountered in clinical care, and to discuss appropriate nursing interventions.

CHAPTER

76

Structure and Function of the Integumentary System

Objectives

76.1 Describe the structure and function of the following three layers of the skin: (1) epidermal (epidermis), (2) dermal (dermis), and (3) subcutaneous (subcutaneous fat).

76.2 Describe the structure and function of the following epidermal appendages: eccrine and apocrine sweat units, sebaceous glands, hair, and nails.

76.3 Discuss the effects of normal aging on the skin.

Facilitating Student Learning

CLASSROOM

Review Activity

- Ask students to review skin, hair, and nail care in a fundamentals or basic nursing text.

Class Assignments

- Assign students to complete the Student Worksheets for Chapter 76 in the Study Guide.
- Assign students to learn the definitions of terms listed in Table 76-1 of the text.
- Ask students to read Greene, et al.: Acquired precursors of cutaneous malignant melanoma: The familial dysplastic nevus syndrome. *New England Journal of Medicine, 31*(2), pp. 91–97, January 10, 1985. This article contains excellent photographs of the lesions that represent the most common, best characterized precursors to malignant melanoma that have been identified.

Lecture/Discussion

- Lead a class discussion on integumentary changes through the life span. Assign a student from each group to develop a teaching plan for people in an age group prone to a particular integumentary problem and to share the highlights of their plan with the class.

Transparency

- 169(T)—Structure of the Skin

CHAPTER

77

Assessment of Clients with Integumentary Disorders

OBJECTIVES

77.1 Obtain a thorough health history, including pertinent past history as well as current abnormalities or problems related to an integumentary assessment.

77.2 Use observation and palpation to obtain an accurate physical integumentary assessment.

77.3 Explain in layman's terminology commonly used diagnostic skin procedures.

77.4 Identify biocultural variations in assessing the integumentary system.

Facilitating Student Learning

CLASSROOM

Class Assignments

- Assign students to complete the activities for Chapter 77 in the Study Guide.
- Assign students to learn the definitions of terms listed in Tables 77-2, 77-3, and 77-4 of the text.
- Refer students to the box on Diversity in Healthcare: Biocultural Variations in the Integumentary System" in Chapter 77 of the text for an excellent discussion of normal and abnormal variations.

Lecture/Discussion

- Color slides showing clinical manifestations of skin disorders make the discussion more interesting.

Transparencies

- 170(T)—Primary Skin Lesions
- 171(T)—Secondary Skin Lesions

Group Activity

- Divide the class into small groups. Ask each group to develop an assessment tool that provides for normal changes in the skin occurring with aging. Then use color slides to differentiate normal from abnormal skin changes.

CLINICAL

Skills Laboratory

- Assign pairs of students to practice integumentary assessment. Refer them to the section on past health history in the textbook to assist them with taking a history relevant to a dermatologic assessment.

Clinical Site Activities

- Ask students to complete an integumentary assessment on the people to whom they are assigned in clinical.
- Assign students on a rotational basis to a dermatology clinic to observe diagnostic skin procedures.

Clinical Conference Activities

- Ask students to share their findings from the skin assessments (history and physical) that they performed on their assigned clients.
- Ask students who were assigned to a dermatology clinic to report on the diagnostic skin procedures they observed, including exactly what was done, the purpose of the procedure, and the postprocedure teaching for the client.

CHAPTER

78

Nursing Care of Clients with Integumentary Disorders

Objectives

78.1 Discuss common dermatologic topical therapies as to action and nursing interventions.

78.2 Describe the purpose and possible complications of ultraviolet light treatment.

78.3 Discuss the psychosocial aspects of skin disorders and associated nursing implications.

78.4 Describe inflammatory skin conditions, in general, as to pathophysiology and etiology, and appropriate nursing and medical interventions.

78.5 Give examples of inflammatory skin conditions (pruritus, eczema/dermatitis, psoriasis, acne, and pemphigus).

78.6 Describe the risk factors, pathophysiology, and four stages of pressure ulcers.

78.7 Discuss medical and nursing interventions for the client with pressure ulcers.

78.8 Describe skin infections and infestations, in general, as to pathophysiology and etiology, and appropriate nursing and medical interventions.

78.9 Give some examples of skin infections (bacterial, fungal, viral, parasitic).

78.10 Describe common nail disorders, in general, as to pathophysiology and etiology, and appropriate nursing and medical interventions.

78.11 Discuss the following specific premalignant and malignant skin conditions as to pathophysiology and etiology, and appropriate nursing and medical interventions: actinic keratosis, basal cell carcinoma, squamous cell carcinoma, malignant melanoma, mycosis fungoides, and Kaposi's sarcoma.

78.12 Outline specific ways to protect the skin from sunlight.

78.13 Teach the client skin self-examination.

Facilitating Student Learning

CLASSROOM

Review Activity

- Ask students to review skin, hair, and nail care in a fundamentals or basic nursing text.

Class Assignment

- Assign students to complete the Study Guide activities for Chapter 78.

Lecture/Discussion

- Discuss the major types of integumentary disorders. Choose examples of each type and discuss pathophysiology and etiology, medical and surgical interventions, and nursing diagnoses with appropriate nursing interventions for each diagnosis. Use a series of slides to present pictorial clinical cases when discussing examples of each type of integumentary disorder.
- Discuss the topic of pressure ulcers and include specific nursing interventions to prevent and treat the condition. Stress the importance of nutritional assessment and management.

Transparencies

- 172(T)—Basal Cell Carcinoma
- 173(T)—Squamous Cell Carcinoma
- 174(T)—Nodular Melanoma

Group Activity

- Divide the class into small groups. Ask each group to develop a teaching plan for people in a particular age group who are prone to a specific integumentary problem; i.e., acne among adolescents or fungal infections among immunosuppressed people.

Guest Speaker

- Invite a dermatologist to discuss the medical management of common integumentary disorders.

CLINICAL

Skills Laboratory

- Arrange for students to practice applying various topical medications and protective dressings.

Clinical Site Activities

- In cooperation with community health faculty, arrange for the student groups to implement their teaching plans to appropriate community groups (see Group Activities).
- Arrange for students to spend some time in a dermatology clinic. If possible, assign students to a clinical nurse specialist or nurse practitioner in that area.
- Assign students in the acute care facility to provide nursing care for clients with integumentary disorders. Ask students to use the appropriate nursing process plans in this chapter and individualize the plans as necessary.
- Expect students to use the Braden Scale to assess their clients in the clinical area. Refer them to Figure 78-6 in the text.

Clinical Conference Activities

- Ask students to share the nursing process plans that they used during the clinical week. Point out commonalties.
- Ask students to try the following "inactivity" at home: Stay in one position (either sitting or lying) for one hour. Discuss their reactions and the nursing research related to the frequency of repositioning clients. Refer them to the Nursing Research box in Chapter 78 of the text.

CHAPTER

79

Nursing Care of Clients with Burns

OBJECTIVES

79.1 Discuss the etiology of burns by describing four categories of burn injuries.

79.2 Identify specific areas to address when planning strategies to prevent burns.

79.3 Describe the systemic effects of burns.

79.4 Describe the effects of carbon monoxide and smoke poisoning.

79.5 List the factors determining burn severity.

79.6 Describe the major categories of burn depth.

79.7 Assess burn size by the "Rule of Nines" technique.

79.8 Describe the Berkow method of determining burn size.

79.9 Discuss how burn location, the medical history and age of the client, and mechanism of injury affect burn severity.

79.10 Discuss appropriate interventions during the emergent phase for the following types of burns: thermal, chemical, and electrical.

79.11 Identify nursing diagnoses common for burned clients.

79.12 Discuss specific nursing interventions, including assessment, appropriate for each of the above nursing diagnoses.

79.13 Describe airway management and oxygen therapy for the client with burns.

79.14 Discuss fluid resuscitation in the first 24 hours and second 24 hours following burn injury.

79.15 Describe management of the client with a circumferential burn.

79.16 Identify basic principles of infection control.

79.17 Discuss hydrotherapy as to purpose, advantages and disadvantages, and nursing considerations.

79.18 Describe the major methods of debridement as to purpose, and advantages and disadvantages.

79.19 Discuss topical therapy as to purpose, advantages and disadvantages, and nursing considerations of specific examples.

79.20 Differentiate between the two methods of burn wound management: (1) open, and (2) closed.

79.21 Discuss care of the skin graft and the donor site.

79.22 Differentiate among the main types of biologic dressings and synthetic dressings.

79.23 Describe the aggressive nutritional support necessary for the client with burns.

79.24 Discuss pharmacologic and nonpharmacologic methods of pain management.

79.25 Describe the psychosocial reactions typical of burned clients.

79.26 Demonstrate correct methods of positioning to prevent contractures.

Facilitating Student Learning

CLASSROOM

Review Activity

- Ask students to review the fire and safety policies and emergency procedures for the clinical agencies where they will be assigned.

Class Assignments

- Assign students to complete the Study Guide activities for Chapter 79.
- Ask students to survey their homes for fire hazards and to suggest ways to improve the safety of their home environment to prevent fires.

Lecture/Discussion

- Lead a class discussion on fire incidence and prevention.
- Discuss the pathophysiology of the categories of burn depth. Transparency 175(T) may be used.
- Emphasize the factors determining burn severity when discussing assessment of a burned client. Transparency 176(T) may be used.
- Discuss nursing care and treatment for the burned client. Include first aid interventions; emergency room management; airway management; fluid resuscitation; infection control; pain relief; body temperature control; promotion of good nutrition and weight maintenance; prevention of stress ulcer, compartment syndrome, and contractures; wound care; debridement and grafting; reconstructive procedures; and rehabilitation. Transparencies 177(M), 178(M), and 179(M) may be used.
- Discuss the psychosocial impact of serious burns and nursing interventions that are helpful.

Transparencies

- 175(T)—Burn Depth
- 176(T)—The Rule of Nines
- 177(M)—Mobility Exercises Following Burns
- 178(M)—Facial Edema Following Burn Injury
- 179(M)—Escharotomy

Guest Speakers

- Invite the environmental safety officer or person in charge of fire prevention and safety within the clinical agency to discuss specific fire safety policies and procedures.
- Invite a clinical nurse specialist from the emergency department to discuss first aid and emergency treatment for the burned client.
- Invite a clinical nurse specialist who works in a burn unit to discuss management of the burned client during the acute phase.
- Invite members of the burn team to discuss rehabilitation of the burned client. Members of the burn rehabilitation team may include a nurse, social worker, nutritionist, psychologist, occupational therapist, physical therapist, and physician.

CLINICAL

Skills Laboratory

- Ask students to practice mobility exercises useful for clients who are rehabilitating following burns.

Clinical Site Activities

- Arrange for students to provide nursing care for burned clients in various stages of therapy. Students may be assigned to the emergency department, surgical intensive care unit, acute burn unit, burn clinic, and rehabilitation unit. Because of the nature of the injuries, students usually will need to be assigned to work with a nurse.
- Arrange for students to accompany clients to the operating room to observe debridement and grafting, and reconstructive and plastic procedures.

Clinical Conference Activities

- Encourage students to discuss their feelings regarding clients with serious burn injuries. Discuss ways the nurse can deal with these feelings and the stresses of working in a burn unit.
- Ask students to share the nursing diagnoses and appropriate nursing interventions used in providing care for the burned clients to whom they were assigned. Compare similarities.

CHAPTER

80

Nursing Care of Clients Undergoing Plastic Surgery

Objectives

80.1 Differentiate between the purposes of aesthetic plastic surgery and reconstructive surgery.

80.2 Differentiate between expectations of clients having aesthetic plastic surgery and those having reconstructive surgery.

80.3 List the basic principles of plastic surgery.

80.4 Discuss how body image is an important consideration when providing care for clients experiencing plastic surgery.

80.5 Outline the following common plastic surgical procedures by including the purpose, brief description of the procedure, and potential complications: rhytidectomy, blepharoplasty, rhinoplasty, and lipectomy.

80.6 Differentiate among the types of grafts used in reconstructive surgery.

80.7 Discuss nursing assessment and interventions for a client with a recent skin graft or tissue transfer that focus on promoting capillary formation.

80.8 Describe laser treatment used in plastic surgery.

80.9 Explain in general terms types of reconstructive breast surgical procedures.

80.10 Discuss postoperative nursing care specific for a client undergoing reconstructive breast surgery.

80.11 Describe assessment findings characteristic of facial fractures.

80.12 Discuss types of facial fractures and stabilization procedures.

80.13 Discuss general nursing intervention for the client with facial fractures.

80.14 Discuss general nursing intervention for the client with facial lacerations.

80.15 Discuss immediate care of a client following traumatic amputation.

80.16 Describe in general terms replantation surgery.

80.17 Discuss nursing intervention for the client following replantation.

Facilitating Student Learning

CLASSROOM

Class Assignment

- Assign students to complete the activities in the Study Guide for Chapter 80.

Lecture/Discussion

- Show slides of clients pre- and postoperatively to illustrate the benefits of the major types of plastic surgery. Emphasize the importance of considering the concept of body image when planning care for clients undergoing plastic surgery.
- Discuss briefly the surgical technique of tissue transfer to help students understand the importance of nursing interventions which are aimed toward ensuring that tissue moved during surgery remains viable. Use Transparency 180(T) when discussing arterialized skin flaps.
- Refer students to the nursing care plan in Chapter 80 of the text when discussing nursing interventions specific to pre- and postoperative wound care.
- Discuss the current ruling from the Food and Drug Administration regarding breast implant surgery for augmentation and reconstruction.
- Discuss pre- and postoperative care for the client with facial fractures.
- Emphasize the necessity of holistic assessment when discussing nursing intervention following replantation to prevent all attention from being focused on the reimplanted part. These clients often undergo long surgical procedures while under general anesthesia and thus may be more prone to respiratory complications postoperatively.

Transparency

- 180(T)—Arterialized Omental Skin Flap

Guest Speaker

- Invite a plastic surgeon to discuss surgical advances and ways nurses can help ensure that the expected results of the surgery are achieved.

Group Activity

- Divide the class into small groups and ask each group to develop a nursing care plan for clients experiencing one of the following types of plastic surgical procedures: blepharoplasty, lipectomy, rhytidectomy, rhinoplasty, postmastectomy breast reconstruction, and reduction mammoplasty.

CLINICAL

Clinical Site Activities

- Arrange for students to provide perioperative care for clients undergoing plastic surgery.
- Assign students to the surgery clinic or a plastic surgeon's office for at least part of a day so they may observe pre- and postoperative progress of clients experiencing plastic surgery.

Clinical Conference Activities

- Ask students to share their care plans developed during group activity (see Group Activities) and any they used during clinical.
- Discuss psychosocial considerations and ask students to share how the clients they observed were adjusting to changes in body image. Discuss nursing interventions that facilitated the adjustment.

CHAPTER

81

Structure and Function of the Reproductive System

OBJECTIVES

81.1 Identify key structures of the male and female reproductive systems.

81.2 Discuss key functions of the male and female reproductive systems.

Facilitating Student Learning

CLASSROOM

Review Activities

- Assign students to review the structure and function of the female and male reproductive systems in this chapter.
- Suggest students answer questions in the Study Guide as a means of verifying their knowledge about structure and function of the female and male reproductive system.

Transparencies

- 181(T)—Organs of Female Reproductive System
- 182(T)—Breast and Mammary Glands (from Jarvis, C. *Physical Examination and Health Assessment*. Philadelphia: W.B. Saunders Co. 1992.)
- 183(T)—Hormonal Regulation of Female Reproductive Functions
- 184(T)—Structures in the Male Reproductive System
- 185(T)—Hormonal Regulation of Testicular Function

CHAPTER

82

Assessment of Clients with Reproductive Disorders

OBJECTIVES

82.1 Identify key elements of a comprehensive gynecologic assessment.

82.2 Describe diagnostic tests used for women with gynecologic disorders.

82.3 Examine key elements of a health assessment for men with reproductive disorders.

82.4 Describe diagnostic tests used for men with disorders of the reproductive system.

82.5 Discuss primary and secondary prevention related to reproductive disorders.

Facilitating Student Learning

CLASSROOM

REVIEW ACTIVITY

- Assign students to review the structure and function of the male and female reproductive systems in Chapter 81.

LECTURE/DISCUSSION

- Focus a student discussion on the impact of gynecologic problems for women and nursing approaches that promote women's satisfaction with their healthcare.
- Discuss components of the gynecologic history and physical examination.
- Discuss the nurse's role in teaching breast self-examination.
- Discuss gynecologic diagnostic procedures and tests. Emphasize the nurse's role during the procedure.
- Discuss elements of the male reproductive/urinary system history and physical examination.
- Emphasize approaches to clients having an examination of their reproductive systems that will be supportive, help decrease their embarrassment and fears, and help maintain their dignity.
- Discuss various diagnostic procedures used when men have reproductive tract disorders.
- Discuss testicular self-examination.
- Emphasize primary and secondary prevention teaching in the area of reproductive disorders.

TRANSPARENCIES

- 186(T)—Sexual Health Assessment
- 187(T)—Assessment of Axillary Lymph Nodes
- 188(T)—Self-Examination of the Female Breasts and Axillae

CLINICAL

SKILLS LABORATORY

- Pair students and have them take a gynecological history on each other.
- Assign students to practice preparing a woman for a gynecological examination. Have a third student "critique" the preparation and make suggestions on how the process could be improved.
- Pair students and have them take a male reproductive system history on each another.

CLINICAL SITE ACTIVITIES

- Assign students to spend the day in a gynecology clinic or physician's office. Have them prepare ahead of time a general nursing care plan focusing on increasing the woman's comfort and understanding of the procedures.
- Assign students to a clinic where men are receiving treatment for reproductive disorders. Have them focus on components of assessment for reproductive disorders.
- As appropriate, encourage students to include teaching their clients testicular self-examination or breast self-examination in their teaching plans.

CLINICAL CONFERENCE ACTIVITIES

- Focus the students' discussion on the interventions they found helpful to the women during the procedures and interventions that did not seem to help relieve discomfort.
- Have students share their experiences with assessing clients with reproductive system disorders.
- Focus discussion on techniques that helped put the clients at ease and questioning techniques that enhanced collection of data.
- As appropriate, assign students to complete a focused history and physical of clients with reproductive disorders.

CHAPTER

83

Nursing Care of Men with Reproductive Disorders

Objectives

83.1 Identify assessment areas pertinent to males with reproductive disturbances.

83.2 Discuss disorders of infertility and impotence and their medical, surgical, and nursing management.

83.3 Discuss disorders of the prostate and their medical, surgical, and nursing management.

83.4 Discuss medical, surgical, and nursing management for the client with testicular disorders.

83.5 Define penile, scrotal, reproductive duct, and seminal vesical disorders.

Facilitating Student Learning

CLASSROOM

Review Activities

- Suggest students review structure and functions of the reproductive and urinary tract in Chapter 81.
- Suggest students review assessment of clients with reproductive and urinary disorders in Chapter 82.
- Assign students to review the process for teaching testicular self-examination in Chapter 82.

Lecture/Discussion

- Discuss psychosocial and cultural factors that may inhibit men from seeking healthcare for reproductive disorders.
- Discuss disorders of the prostate and medical, surgical, and perioperative nursing management of these disorders.
- Discuss the nurse's health teaching role for men at risk from environmental, occupational, and pharmacologic agents that may affect the reproductive system.
- Discuss the incidence, psychosocial implications, and treatment for male infertility.
- Discuss the causes and treatment of erectile dysfunction.
- Discuss the impact of and treatment for infertility and impotence.
- Discuss testicular cancer and its medical, surgical, and nursing management.
- Emphasize to students the importance of teaching their male clients testicular self-examination.
- Review with students the clinical pathways for TURP and simple orchiectomy in Appendix D.

Transparencies

- 189(T)—Penile Prostheses
- 190(T)—Potential Complications of Benign Prostatic Hypertrophy. (From Smith, D.R. *General Urology* [11th ed.]. Los Altos, Calif.: Lange Medical Publications, 1994.)
- 191(T)—Types of Catheters
- 192(T)—Surgical Approaches to the Prostate
- 193(T)—Disorders of the Testicles
- 194(T)—Vasectomy

Guest Speaker

- Invite a pharmacist to discuss ways men can decrease the sexual and reproductive side effects of certain medications.

CLINICAL

Skills Laboratory

- Pair students and have them role play taking a history related to the male reproductive system. Suggest the students practice techniques that will put the person at ease.
- Show students various catheters, irrigation of catheters, and drainage systems.
- Review with students catheterization of the male client.

Clinical Site Activities

- Assign students to care for males who are hospitalized with reproductive disorders.
- Assist students to assess the client with a catheter.

Clinical Conference Activities

- Focus the students' discussion on how they were or were not able to ease their own and their client's embarrassment when discussing reproductive disorders. For the students who were not able to ease the discomfort, discuss ways the problem could be handled in the future.
- Work with students to develop a nursing care plan for the client with urethral and suprapubic catheters, postoperative transurethral resection, suprapubic prostatectomy, or retropubic prostatectomy.

Critical Points to Emphasize

Infertility

- Incidence
- Causes
- Normal sperm count
- Clinical manifestations
- Diagnostic findings
- Pretesticular, testicular, and post-testicular causes
- Medical management
- Nursing management: primary prevention, assessment, teaching about diagnostic tests and use of testosterone patches, referral to counseling or support groups

Benign Prostatic Hypertrophy

- Incidence
- Etiology
- Risk factors
- Pathophysiology
- Clinical manifestations
- Diagnostic findings
- Surgical management: differentiate among various surgical procedures
- Complications
- Nursing management: nursing history and explanation of procedures, support, reassurance, assessment for hemorrhage, maintenance of drains, maintenance of patent catheters, pain control, prevention of constipation, aseptic techniques, teaching about temporary urinary frequency or incontinence, maintaining hydration, teaching home care, and perineal exercises
- Medical management
- Nursing management: assessment, catheterization, teaching about maintaining fluid balance and how to prevent retention and distention

Erectile Dysfunction

- Psychogenic and physiologic dysfunction
- Surgical management
- Nursing management: teaching about use of the prosthesis, pain control, postoperative care
- Medical management: same as for infertility, support client in counseling therapy

Prostate Cancer

- Incidence
- Etiology
- Risk factors
- Pathophysiology
- Clinical manifestations
- Diagnostic tests
- American Cancer Society's early detection recommendations
- Medical management
- Nursing care: care of the client receiving radiation and/or chemotherapy or hormonal therapy
- Surgical management: options
- Nursing management: essentially the same as for TURP adding supportive care for the client with cancer

(Continued)

(Concluded)

Testicular Tumors

- Incidence
- Etiology
- ACS early detection recommendations
- Testicular self-examination
- Risk factors
- Pathophysiology
- Clinical manifestations
- Diagnostic findings
- Surgical management: options
- Nursing management: assessment, teaching client about potential complications, pain control, postoperative care
- Medical management: radiation and chemotherapy
- Nursing management: assessment, reassurance and support

CHAPTER

84

Nursing Care of Women with Gynecologic Disorders

Objectives

84.1 Discuss menstrual disorders and menopause and their medical, surgical, and nursing management.

84.2 Discuss infectious and inflammatory uterine disorders and their medical, surgical, and nursing management.

84.3 Discuss malignant and nonmalignant tumors of the uterus and their medical, surgical, and nursing management.

84.4 Discuss other disorders of the uterus and their medical, surgical, and nursing management.

84.5 Discuss ovarian disorders and their medical, surgical, and nursing management.

84.6 Discuss vaginal disorders and their medical, surgical, and nursing management.

84.7 Discuss disorders of the vulva and their medical, surgical, and nursing management.

84.8 Define other gynecologic cancers.

Facilitating Student Learning

CLASSROOM

Review Activities

- Encourage students to review Chapter 81 on the structure and function of the female reproductive system.
- Have students review Chapter 82 on assessment of the female reproductive system.

Lecture/Discussion

- Discuss disorders of menstruation and menopause. Assign students to bring articles from lay literature as input for the discussion.
- Discuss common disorders of the uterus, vagina, cervix, and vulva.
- Emphasize to students aspects of teaching for women who have common disorders uterus, vagina, cervix, and vulva.
- Review the use of pharmacologic agents in treatment of vaginal infections.
- Facilitate class discussion on nursing care for the physical and emotional effects on the client undergoing cryotherapy, vulvectomy, and hysterectomy.
- Discuss manifestations and routes of spread of pelvic inflammatory disease (PID).
- Discuss the condition and etiology of endometriosis. Transparency 196(T) may be useful in this discussion.
- Facilitate a class discussion on nursing diagnoses and interventions for a client undergoing medical or surgical treatment for endometriosis.
- Discuss the various nonmalignant pelvic masses.
- Discuss fistulas of the vagina and nursing and medical interventions.
- Differentiate among the three degrees of uterine prolapse and discuss cystoceles and rectoceles.
- Focus student discussion on nursing care for clients having medical or surgical treatments for uterine prolapse and cystocele and rectocele.
- Focus a student discussion on the psychological and physical impact of gynecologic cancer.
- Emphasize the nurse's role in assessing and intervening for psychological and physical responses to gynecologic cancer.
- Discuss the incidence of primary vaginal cancer and the role of diethylstilbestrol (DES).
- Discuss diagnosis and surgical treatment for early and advanced vaginal cancer.
- Discuss the possible effects of vaginal surgery on sexual function and nursing interventions.
- Emphasize common nursing diagnoses, interventions, and follow-up care for clients undergoing treatment for cervical or endometrial cancer.
- Discuss the spread of, assessment findings on, and interventions for ovarian cancer.
- Organize a student debate for and against the use of hormone replacement therapy for menopausal women.
- Organize a student discussion on ethnic and cultural differences in attitudes and practices related to aspects of female reproduction.

Transparencies

- 195(T)—Routes of Spread of PID
- 196(T)—Sites of Endometriosis
- 197(T)—Locations of Uterine Leiomyomas (Fibroids)
- 198(T)—Sites of Benign Gynecologic Lesions
- 199(T)—Vaginal Fistulas
- 200(T)—Displaced Positions of the Uterus
- 201(T)—Uterine Prolapse
- 202(T)—Cystocele and Rectocele
- 203(T)—Radical Vulvectomy

Guest Speaker

- Invite a woman who has had gynecologic surgery to share her experiences with students. Focus part of the discussion on interventions nurses could implement to increase women's physical and emotional comfort.

CLINICAL

Clinical Site Activities

- Assign students to care for clients hospitalized with nonmalignant or malignant gynecologic disorders and to develop nursing diagnoses and interventions.
- Assign students to accompany clients to surgery who are having gynecologic surgery. Encourage the students to assess for and intervene in the client's emotional and physiological needs.
- Assign students to care for clients who are undergoing medical treatment for gynecologic cancers. Encourage students to include safety precautions for either the chemotherapy or radiation implant in their plan of care.

Clinical Conference Activities

- Focus student discussion of physical and emotional responses they assessed in their clients undergoing gynecologic surgery. Work in small groups to develop nursing interventions to care for these clients.
- Facilitate a discussion of safety measures when caring for a client with a radium implant.
- Work with students to develop teaching plans that focus on primary prevention and/or early detection for cervical cancer, PID, endometrial cancer, vaginitis, vulvitis, and vulvar cancer.

Critical Points to Emphasize

Dysmenorrhea

- Differentiate primary and secondary
- Prostaglandin role
- Differentiate from premenstrual syndrome (PMS)
- Etiology
- Pathophysiology
- Clinical course
- Medical management: use of nonpharmacologic remedies, contraception, exercise, prostaglandin synthesis inhibitors
- Nursing management: education, support, nutrition, exercise, rest and sleep, and assess stress levels

Pelvic Inflammatory Disease

- Pathophysiology
- Clinical manifestations
- Risk factors
- Risk for infertility
- Primary prevention
- Medical management
- Surgical management
- Nursing management: support, education about hygiene measures, safe sexual practices, nutrition, rest, sleep, and exercise

Menopause

- Review physiology
- Compare natural menopause with surgical menopause
- Manifestations
- Medical management: hormone replacement therapy (HRT), contraindications for HRT treatment for atrophic vaginitis
- Nursing management: education about managing hot flashes, support, education about HRT, self-care education about vaginal dryness, osteoporosis, urinary tract infections (UTIs), and Kegel exercises

Endometriosis

- Etiology
- Risk factors
- Pathophysiology
- Clinical manifestations
- Medical management: focus on medications
- Surgical management
- Nursing management: education about disorder, medications, and symptom management

Endometrial Cancer

- Incidence
- Etiology
- Risk factors
- Primary prevention
- Pathophysiology
- Clinical manifestations
- Diagnostic findings, accuracy of Pap smear
- Medical management
- Surgical management: types of hysterectomies
- Nursing management: preoperative teaching; understanding of loss of reproductive capacity; postoperative care; maintenance of urinary catheter; prevention of constipation; support for loss, depending on type of hysterectomy and age; may have onset of menopause; will not be candidate for HRT; discharge teaching about abdominal strengthening exercises; avoid heavy lifting and activities that will increase pelvic congestion; avoid sexual intercourse for about six weeks; report signs of infections

Ovarian Cancer

- Incidence
- Risk factors
- Primary prevention
- Early detection
- Pathophysiology
- Clinical manifestations
- Surgical management
- Medical management
- Nursing care (see nursing care above for client having a hysterectomy)

Cervical Cancer

- Incidence
- Pathophysiology
- Risk factors
- Clinical manifestations
- Diagnostic procedures: Pap smear, Schiller's, cold conization, cryosurgery
- Medical management: irradiation
- Nursing management: care of the client having irradiation, cervical implants, information about managing vaginal changes, emphasis on follow-up care
- Surgical management: options
- Nursing management: education about type of surgery, psychological support, personal hygiene, potential need for adaptations in intercourse methods

Vulvar Cancer

- Risk factors
- Primary prevention
- Early detection
- Etiology
- Pathophysiology
- Clinical manifestations
- Medical management
- Nursing management: supportive through diagnostic period, treatment for symptoms
- Surgical management: surgical options
- Nursing management: psychological support; preoperative preparation: enema, douche, Foley catheter; education about surgery; postoperative: maintenance of drains, leg exercises, perineal care, incisional infection prevention methods, monitor urination and bowel movements, impact on sexuality, discharge teaching

CHAPTER

85

Nursing Care of Clients with Breast Disorders

Objectives

85.1 Discuss breast cancer and its medical, surgical, and nursing management.

85.2 Describe benign breast disorders and their medical and nursing management.

Facilitating Student Learning

CLASSROOM

Review Activities

- Encourage students to review normal structure and function of the breast in Chapter 81 and assessment of the breast in Chapter 82.
- Encourage students to review the procedure for mammography and breast self-examination (BSE).

Lecture/Discussion

- Emphasize the nurse's responsibilities in teaching about breast lesions, the risk factors, early detection techniques, and the American Cancer Society's recommendations for frequency of early detection techniques.
- Discuss breast cancer incidence, the change in breast cancer statistics since the text was published, and breast cancer risk factors.
- Discuss histopathologic types of breast cancer, initial assessment findings, locations of cancer in the breast, and prognosis.
- Discuss staging and grading of breast cancer.
- Explain various parameters for determining breast cancer prognosis and tests for proliferative activity.
- Describe the surgical options for breast cancer.
- Encourage students to help identify nursing diagnoses and interventions for women experiencing breast cancer.
- Using Transparency 208(T), describe postmastectomy exercises.
- Discuss the uses of radiation therapy with breast cancer.
- Discuss misunderstandings people may have about radiation.
- Discuss teaching/learning for women undergoing radiation for breast cancer.
- Explain the estrogen receptor assay test and its implications for hormonal treatment.
- Discuss hormonal manipulation methods.
- Discuss the uses of chemotherapy for treating breast cancer and common chemotherapy agents used.
- Discuss nursing care for women receiving chemotherapy for breast cancer.
- Discuss the course of metastasis with breast cancer and complications that may occur.
- Discuss the benign breast disorders and their treatments.
- Review with students the clinical pathway for mastectomy in Appendix D.

Transparencies

- 205(T)—Risk Factors for Breast Cancer (Adapted from Kelsey, J.L., & Gammon, M.D. The epidemiology of breast cancer. Calif: *A Cancer Journal for Clinicians, 41*[3], 1991, p. 157.)
- 206(T)—Frequency of Occurrence of Breast Cancer According to Location
- 207(T)—Clinical Staging of Breast Cancer
- 208(T)—Postmastectomy Exercises

Guest Speaker

- Invite a volunteer from Reach for Recovery to explain to students her role with women who have had mastectomies.

CLINICAL

Clinical Site Activities

- Assign students to care for women undergoing tests for breast cancer.
- Encourage students to include the teaching of breast self-examination in their care plans as appropriate.
- Assign students to care for women being treated medically and/or surgically for breast cancer and to develop nursing diagnoses and interventions to direct care.

Clinical Conference Activity

- Facilitate a student discussion on physical and psychosocial nursing diagnoses and interventions for women with mastectomies.

Critical Points to Emphasize

Breast Cancer	Fibrocystic Breasts
• Public attitudes • Incidence • Etiology • Risk factors • Primary prevention and early detection measures • Pathophysiology: description of different histopathologic types • Clinical manifestations • Diagnostic findings • Surgical options and breast reconstruction • Nursing management: assessment, identification of risk factors, support and reassurance, information about treatment options, preoperative teaching, identification of coping mechanisms, postoperative care, assessment for body image and sexuality problems, information about prosthesis or reconstruction, maintenance of drains, support adjusting to wound, teaching about arm edema, exercises, prevention of infection, and Reach for Recovery consultation • Medical management: radiation therapy, chemotherapy, hormone therapy, and bone marrow transplant • Nursing management: teaching about chemotherapy, radiation and symptom management, nutrition, fatigue, and support for grieving • Metastatic breast cancer • Breast cancer in men	• Incidence • Etiology • Assessment findings • Treatment: breast support with fitted brassiere, hot and cold applications, analgesics, diuretics, reducing dietary intake of methylxanthines, vitamin E, use of androgens

CHAPTER

86

Nursing Care of Clients with Sexually Transmitted Diseases

Objectives

86.1 Examine the overall concept of sexually transmitted diseases (STDs) and medical and nursing management.

86.2 Discuss common sexually transmitted diseases and their medical and nursing management.

86.3 Describe the remaining, less common sexually transmitted diseases.

Facilitating Student Learning

CLASSROOM

CLASS ASSIGNMENT

- Assign students to complete definitions and questions in Chapter 86 of the Study Guide.

LECTURE/DISCUSSION

- Emphasize to students the importance of a nonjudgmental approach when working with clients with STDs.
- Emphasize the primary role of the nurse as teacher when working with clients with STDs.
- Engage students in a discussion about possible reasons for the increase in STDs.
- Discuss with students primary prevention approaches for different age and gender groups.
- Discuss with students various pharmacologic agents used to treat STDs, their potential side effects, and important aspects for client teaching.
- Discuss laboratory tests used in the diagnosis of STDs.
- Emphasize the implications for clients of untreated STDs.
- Develop with students a list of interview questions appropriate for clients with suspected or diagnosed STDs.

TRANSPARENCY

- 204(T)—Sexually Transmitted Diseases

CLINICAL

SKILLS LABORATORY

- Assign students in pairs to practice interviewing a client with an actual or suspected STD using the questions developed in class.

CLINICAL SITE ACTIVITIES

- Assign students to clinics where clients with STDs are treated.
- Assign students to review laboratory findings, to assist with client interviews, to carry out prescribed treatments, and to develop and implement client teaching.

CLINICAL CONFERENCE ACTIVITIES

- Have students share their experiences at clinics.
- Facilitate a discussion on the interviews students completed and the approaches that yielded the most information from clients.
- Work with students to develop one or two nursing care plans based on the plans they developed, implemented, and evaluated.

Critical Points to Emphasize

Sexually Transmitted Diseases

- Common characteristics
- Identify sexually transmitted diseases
- Prevalence
- Mandatory reporting
- Increased incidence
- Etiology
- Pathophysiology
- Risk factors
- Primary prevention
- Manifestations of common STDs
- Diagnostics
- Medical management: antibiotics of choice
- Confidentiality
- Nursing management: physical assessment and sexual history; teaching about transmission, prevention, and treatment of STDs; correction of misconceptions about STDs; effective use of mechanical barriers (condoms); reduce anxiety; provide support; and have a nonjudgmental attitude

CHAPTER

87

Substance Abuse

Objectives

87.1 Discuss the heath problem of substance abuse.

87.2 Define terms related to substance abuse.

87.3 Discuss theories about the causes of substance abuse.

87.4 Describe assessment for and the effects of psychoactive substances.

87.5 Discuss the nursing care of clients with substance abuse.

87.6 Discuss the effects of use and abuse of alcohol.

87.7 Discuss the effects of use and abuse of stimulants.

87.8 Discuss the effects of use and abuse of cannabis.

87.9 Discuss the ethical issues of the chemically impaired co-worker.

Facilitating Student Learning

CLASSROOM

Class Assignment

- Assign students to complete Chapter 87 in the Study Guide before class.

Lecture/Discussion

- Have students complete a self-awareness instrument that provides the students with insight about personal values and beliefs about substance abuse. The Seaman-Mannello Scale and the National Council on Alcoholism and Drug Dependence Scale are examples of these instruments. Provide time for the students to express their feelings concerning substance abuse. This topic is often an emotionally charged subject that elicits a variety of responses. There may be several students who have had experiences (either personal or family members) with substance abuse.
- Assign students to write a one-page reflective paper on their attitudes and feelings about substance abuse.
- Discuss the biologic, psychological, and sociocultural frameworks for explaining addictive behavior.
- Discuss the combination of factors that help explain the development of substance abuse or dependence.
- Discuss the *Diagnostic and Statistical Manual of Mental Disorders (DSM IV)* definition and classifications of substance abuse.
- Discuss the terminology related to substance abuse (Table 87-1).
- Discuss the behavior changes, tolerance, physical and psychological dependence, and withdrawal involved with the 11 types of substances in the DSM IV (use Tables 87-2 and 87-4 as references).
- Discuss alcohol/drug interactions and teaching/learning that needs to accompany medications that interact with alcohol. The article by C.E. Northrop, "Don't overlook discharge teaching about drugs," *Nursing '86, 16*(11):43, can be used to emphasize the legal responsibilities regarding teaching.
- Discuss caring for the substance abuse client in the acute care setting.
- Discuss the effects of substance abuse on people requiring surgery.
- Using some of the nursing diagnoses suggested in Box 87-3 of the textbook, focus a student discussion on developing interventions for the nursing diagnoses. When the nursing diagnoses involve long-term specialized treatments that would not be feasible in the acute care setting, assist the students to identify referral resources.
- Emphasize the incidence of substance abuse with nurses. Use Box 87-8 and Ethical Issues in Nursing, What Ethical Issues Surround Your Relationship to an Impaired Nurse?

Guest Speakers

- Invite a person from the community who can discuss resources for alcohol and drug treatment programs.
- Invite a person from the State Board of Nursing or other informed person to discuss with students the problems of nurse addiction, licensing implications, and treatment programs.

CLINICAL

Clinical Site Activities

- Assign students to care for a client with alcohol or drug dependence. Encourage students to use information from the textbook on the physical and psychosocial problems associated with alcohol or drug dependence to guide their assessment and explain findings.
- Encourage students to use Box 87-2 and Table 87-3 in the textbook to guide history taking related to alcohol and drug use. If students identify problems with alcohol or drug use, assist them to identify appropriate referrals.
- If possible, assign students to visit different drug and alcohol treatment facilities in the community.

Clinical Conference Activities

- Assign students to report on the treatment facilities they visited, and facilitate a discussion on the similarities and differences in treatment approaches.
- Have the students who cared for clients with drug and alcohol dependence discuss their physical and psychosocial assessment findings, medical treatment, and nursing diagnoses and interventions.

CHAPTER

88

Basic Concepts of Emergency Care

OBJECTIVES

88.1 Discuss situations that hospitals, nurses, and physicians are required to report to appropriate agencies.

88.2 Explain the proper handling of evidence, bullets, and specimens.

88.3 Discuss laws governing client admission and transfer.

88.4 Discuss initial nursing assessment, triage categories, documentation, secondary nursing assessments, and discharge teaching in the emergency department.

88.5 Discuss death and dying in emergency settings.

88.6 Discuss the religious, ethical, and legal issues concerning organ donation.

Facilitating Student Learning

CLASSROOM

Classroom Assignments

- Assign students to complete Chapter 88 in the Study Guide prior to class.
- Provide students with a list of medications on the crash cart, and ask them to prepare a brief drug card for each medication.

Lecture/Discussion

- Discuss the concept of emergency nursing according to the Emergency Nurses' Association. Refer students to the definition of *emergency nursing* in the text and discuss standards for emergency nursing developed by the Emergency Nurses' Association.
- Discuss the ethical and legal considerations of emergency room care.
- Discuss how the nursing process differs in emergency nursing from other types of nursing.
- Discuss specific needs of the person and significant others in death and dying situations in emergency care settings.
- Discuss the concept of the emergency triage: emergent, urgent, and nonurgent. Use Table 88-1 as a guide.
- Discuss organ donation and organ transplant. Refer to Table 88-2 for the major religions and cultural groups' customs and beliefs.
- Discuss the concept of triage and go over the assessment findings that indicate a high priority for care. Emphasize the importance of looking for injuries that may not be obvious but that may be present because of the type of accident; e.g., a badly contused kidney when the person has costovertebral angle (CVA) pain following an accident, or an injury to the cervical spine when the person has head trauma.
- Discuss the initial nursing assessment. Use the mnemonic AMPLE as a guide for priority health history. Emphasize the importance of a thorough symptom analysis. Use the mnemonic PQRST or OLD CART as examples of a symptom analysis.
- Discuss priority nursing care. Refer to Box 88-1 for assessment findings that indicate a high priority for care.
- Use case studies to discuss assessment and interventions for specific emergencies.
- Discuss the legal implications of emergency care. Sharing some examples from case law makes this more interesting for students.
- Facilitate a discussion about psychosocial and spiritual needs of the client and family in an emergency situation.
- Demonstrate the use of flow sheets to document assessments.
- Discuss various hospital protocols for telephone triage. Use Box 88-2 as a guide.
- Emphasize the importance of careful documentation in the emergency department.

Transparencies

- 214(T)—Cricothyroidotomy
- 215(T)—Esophageal Obturator Airway (Figure 80-3)
- 218(T)—Spine Immobilization Devices (Figure 80-5)

Group Activity

- Review basic CPR and the ABCs of priority assessment and interventions.

Guest Speakers

- Invite a nurse whose specialty is emergency nursing to discuss emergency nursing in the healthcare system.
- Invite a nurse who works with organ donation and transplants to discuss legal and ethical issues related to organ donation.

CLINICAL

Skills Laboratory

- Demonstrate the following emergency equipment: oxygen tank, oral airway, resuscitator bag with mask, pocket mask, esophageal obturator airway (EOA), defibrillator, blood pump, short and long spine boards, Philadelphia collar, and traction splint with ankle hitch. Ask students to return the demonstration on the equipment as appropriate.
- Role play with some students as persons with various injuries and medical conditions necessitating emergency care, so others may practice triage.
- Discuss the use of the crash cart while showing students the contents.
- Design a "mock code" experience for the students.
- Assign students to practice CPR according to current standards of the American Heart Association. If students are not currently certified in basic CPR, assign them to obtain current certification.

Clinical Site Activity

- Ask students to obtain information concerning the legal aspects of emergency nursing as practiced in the emergency department of the hospital in which they are having their clinical experiences.

Clinical Conference Activity

- Invite an organ transplant recipient and an organ donor or an organ donor's family to share personal experiences. Ensure adequate time for sharing and a question-and-answer period.

CHAPTER

89

Nursing Care of Clients with Medical-Surgical Emergencies

Objectives

89.1 Discuss primary assessment and priority nursing interventions in emergency situations.

89.2 Discuss secondary nursing assessments in emergency situations.

89.3 Identify signs and symptoms associated with selected medical-surgical emergencies.

89.4 Describe appropriate medical management and priority discharge teaching of clients with medical-surgical emergencies.

Facilitating Student Learning

CLASSROOM

Class Assignment

- Assign students to complete Chapter 89 in the Study Guide prior to class.

Lecture/Discussion

- Discuss how the nursing process and decision making differs in emergency nursing from other types of nursing.
- Discuss the ABCs (airway, breathing, circulation, cervical spine, and consciousness level) of assessment in an emergency situation.
- Discuss the unique psychosocial needs of the emergent client and significant others.
- List the steps in an initial survey and treatment of a traumatized individual or someone brought to the emergency department with a decreased level of consciousness. Refer students to the Champion trauma score (Table 89-1).
- Make an overhead of the mnemonic "vowel tipps" for clients with altered level of consciousness and discuss each component.
- Demonstrate the use of flow sheets to document assessments.
- Use case studies to discuss assessment and interventions for specific emergencies.
- Discuss common poisonings and their antidotes.
- Facilitate a discussion about psychosocial and spiritual needs of the client and family an emergency situation.
- Discuss the use of tetanus prophylaxis in the emergency situation.
- Emphasize the importance of careful documentation in the emergency department.

Transparencies

- 216(T)—Flail Chest
- 217(M)—Emergency Devices for Tension Pneumothorax

Guest Speakers

- Invite a nurse whose specialty is emergency nursing to discuss emergency nursing in the healthcare system.
- Invite a nurse whose specialty is alleged sexual abuse to discuss the nursing care and follow-up care of alleged sexual abuse victims.

Group Activities

- Divide the class into groups. Give each group a case presentation of an individual needing emergency care and ask the students to develop a care plan to include nursing diagnoses and interventions for continued assessment, appropriate treatment interventions, and evaluation criteria (goals or outcome criteria).
- Assign groups of students to locate or develop a protocol for management of a person with a specific emergency.
- Distribute the same case presentation of a traumatized individual to each group and ask the students to determine the trauma score using the Trauma Score sheet. Lead a class discussion on the results.
- With groups of students serving as teams, have a contest by asking questions concerning information about medications on the crash cart.

CLINICAL

Skills Laboratory

- Design mock emergency room situations using examples in the textbook as a guide.
- Have the students take turns role playing the nurse and the client in as many of the situations as time allows. Allow time to debrief the students, focusing on primary priority assessments and nursing care.
- If your library has videos, interactive videos, or CDs of medical-surgical emergencies, assign students to view preselected emergency situations.

Clinical Site Activities

- Arrange for each student to spend time in an emergency department and with a local mobile emergency care system. Tell the students that they may assist with care at the discretion of the nurse to whom they are assigned, but to understand that they may need to step back into the observer role in many instances. Ask the students to then watch what the nurses do and when there is an opportunity, talk to them about the decisions they made and the priorities they set.
- Ask students to obtain information concerning the legal aspects of emergency nursing as practiced in the emergency department of the hospital in which they are having their clinical experiences.

Clinical Conference Activities

- Invite a person who has experienced a medical or surgical emergency to share how it felt to be suddenly physically vulnerable and the kinds of actions of nurses that helped them feel less anxious and those actions that increased their anxiety.
- Encourage students to discuss their experiences and feelings resulting from their clinical site activities.
- Discuss emergency situations unique or applicable to their community.